ON THE TAKE

On the Take

HOW AMERICA'S COMPLICITY WITH BIG BUSINESS CAN ENDANGER YOUR HEALTH

JEROME P. KASSIRER, M.D.

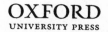

OXFORD
UNIVERSITY PRESS

2005

OXFORD
UNIVERSITY PRESS

OXFORD   NEW YORK

AUCKLAND   BANGKOK   BUENOS AIRES   CAPE TOWN   CHENNAI
DAR ES SALAAM   DELHI   HONG KONG   ISTANBUL   KARACHI   KOLKATA
KUALA LUMPUR   MADRID   MELBOURNE   MEXICO CITY   MUMBAI   NAIROBI
SÃO PAULO   SHANGHAI   TAIPEI   TOKYO   TORONTO

Published by Oxford University Press, Inc.
198 Madison Avenue, New York, New York 10016
www.oup.com

Oxford is a registered trademark of Oxford University Press

Library of Congress Cataloging-in-Publication Data
Kassirer, Jerome P., 1932–
On the take : how medicine's complicity with big business can endanger your
health / by Jerome P. Kassirer.
p. ; cm. Includes bibliographical references and index.
ISBN 0-19-517684-7
1. Physicians—Professional ethics—United States.
2. Pharmaceutical industry—Corrupt practices—United States.
3. Medical ethics—United States.   4. Conflict of interest.   5. Gifts.
[DNLM: 1. Practice Management, Medical—ethics.
2. Conflict of Interest.   3. Physician Incentive Plans—ethics.
4. Physician's Practice Patterns—ethics.   5. Physician's Role.
6. Physician-Patient Relations—ethics. W 50 K188o 2004]
I. Title: How medicine's complicity with big business can endanger your health.
II. Title.
R725.5.K376 2004   174.2'6—dc22 2004012890

1 3 5 7 9 8 6 4 2

Printed in the United States of America
on acid-free paper

to Sheridan

Acknowledgments

I am grateful to dozens, scores, and possibly hundreds of physicians. Many contributed their time, knowledge, and wisdom to help me delve into the kind, extent, and consequences of physicians' collaborations with industry. Many were forthcoming and eager to get the problem exposed. I also interviewed many who were defensive, even angry at the inference that financial conflicts might have influenced their medical decisions. I understand their attitude: because financial arrangements with industry create an impossible-to-resolve dilemma between a doctor's professional role and his or her personal responsibilities, exposure of their conflict is a moral stigmatizer. Interestingly, I also interviewed many others who had no financial conflicts and expressed their moral indignation about the misdeeds of their colleagues who did, yet demurred when I asked to cite their quotes by name. They disappointed me. Financial conflicts of interest invoke strong emotions.

Support from the Josiah Macy Jr. Foundation, the Open Society Institute, and the American Board of Internal Medicine Foundation made the project possible. June Osborn at the Macy Foundation, Gara LaMarche and David Rothman at OSI, and Harry Kimball and Christine Cassel at ABIM deserve special mention for their encouragement. The foundation support made it possible to hire three enthusiastic and outstanding research assistants, Ethan Eddy and Vu Luu from Tufts University School of Medicine and Lisa Olmos from Baylor College of Medicine. Their contributions were both technical and intellectual. I owe a special debt of gratitude to my bosses who created the academic atmosphere and the flexible teaching schedule that allowed me to devote time to the book. They include John T. Harrington, Nicolaos Madias, Michael Rosenblatt, and Deeb Salem at Tufts

University School of Medicine, and David Kessler, Ralph Horwitz, and David Coleman at Yale University School of Medicine. Raymond Tye, an old friend and former patient who is silently behind many medical projects in Boston, provided substantial financial support for my position at Tufts.

Many people enriched my understanding of the subject, debated the pros and cons of relations with industry, read drafts of chapters, provided information, and made invaluable suggestions. They include Elliott Antman, Robert Bass, William Bennett, David Blumenthal, Sandy Bogucki, Robert Bonow, Dawn Bravata, Troyen Brennan, Susan Chimonas, James Cleeman, Jordan Cohen, Douglas Drossman, Thomas Duffy, Peter Eisenberg, Scott Epstein, Mark Feldman, Thomas Finucane, Marshall Folstein, Joanne Foody, Howard Gardner, Lawrence Gartner, Thomas Glynn, Stephen Goldfinger, William Gouveia, William Grossman, Karen Hein, James Herndon, Cora Ho, Jerry Hoffman, Timothy Johnson, Ingrid Katz, Norman Katz, Paul Katz, Ruth Katz, Vincent Kerr, Harry Kimball, Harlan Krumholz, Neil Kurtzman, Andrew Levey, Peter Libby, David Lowance, Kenneth Ludmerer, Eric Mazur, Donald Moore, Carol Nadelson, James Naughton, Joseph Palca, Brian Pereira, Eric Peterson, Robert Reisman, Ellen Relkin, John Ritchie, Marc Rodwin, David Rothman, Harry Selker, David Shriger, Neil Smelser, Robert Steinbrook, Samuel Thier, Dennis Thompson, Robert Utiger, Shaw Warren, Douglas Waud, John Wennberg, James Weyhemeyer, Stephen Winter, and Alexi Wright. Inevitably, this list will be incomplete.

The book covers many aspects of medicine in which I am not an expert, as well as fields such as psychology and sociology. In all these disciplines I relied on the knowledge and advice of many of the above people and others for accuracy and interpretation of information, but in the final analysis any misinterpretations are my own.

I also relied heavily on the outstanding work of several reporters, many of whom have doggedly pursued the well-hidden financial conflicts of physicians for years. They include Liz Kowalczyk at the *Boston Globe*, Andrew Julien and Matthew Kauffman at the *Hartford Courant*, David Willman at the *Los Angeles Times*, Melody Petersen, Kurt Eichenwald, and Gina Kolata at the *New York Times*, Duff Wilson and David Heath at the *Seattle Times*, Jennifer Washburn and Eyal Press of the *Atlantic Monthly*, and Dennis Cauchon at *USA Today*. Melody Petersen deserves special mention because of the extent and excellence of her work.

Special credit goes to Larry Tye, former reporter for the *Boston Globe*. To my delight, Larry became my mentor. He urged me to apply for foundation support and to hire research assistants to help with the work. He pressed me to go beyond a literature survey, to use the techniques of investigative reporting, and to go after substantial fresh material to supplement all that was already available in journals and newspapers. In lunch meetings in Cambridge over many months, he listened patiently to my progress, pushed me hard, and helped me become a fledgling reporter. Theresa Park, my agent, never lost faith in the project, and found it the right home with Oxford University Press, where my superb editor, Timothy Bartlett, improved the book's organization, style, writing, and especially the logic.

The love, support, and unshakable optimism of my children—Amy, Richard, Wendy, Elizabeth, Winston, and Sam—have heightened the many peaks of my career and blunted the occasional valley. I owe them more than they owe me.

Nobody deserves more credit than my wife, Sheridan. Within weeks after I left the *New England Journal of Medicine* in 1999, she began encouraging me to write a book, and her support has been unfailing. Despite her own demanding schedule, she never failed to listen patiently to my daily stories and occasional frustrations. In her "copious free time" she uncomplainingly read and edited the entire book three times. Her integrity, intelligence, tenacity, and her love continue to be an inspiration.

Contents

Introduction

The desire for money is a powerful motivator, and our special brand of capitalism has relied on this incentive to make our country one of the most prosperous in the world. Most doctors eschew any commercial arrangements that might compromise their professional values, yet some have not resisted the buzz of a marketplace that values a profitable bottom line and promises enormous personal wealth. Today the income of many practitioners is several hundred thousand dollars or more, and for some, joining the ranks of academic medicine can be a ticket to great wealth and privilege. Given the expertise of our practitioners and researchers in diagnosing and curing us, and in finding new and better tests and treatments, few of us would begrudge them such wealth as long as we were confident that they are always using their talents and diagnostic tools in our best interests. But are they?

The time has come to ask whether all of the money floating around medicine has created a pattern of corruption. Have the fees that physicians charge given them an incentive to bring patients back to their offices too often or to order too many tests that aren't needed? Or have they skimped on tests if ordering too many shrinks their paycheck? Are they more inclined to order certain expensive drugs or promote certain products because of personal financial relations with some of the drug companies, contrary to patients' best interests?

Most people are accustomed to seeing trinkets bearing drug company names and logos in their doctors' offices, but few are aware that the relations between many doctors and industry run far deeper. Away from the eyes of the public, the pharmaceutical industry captures the loyalty of physicians with gifts and lavish meals, pays them as consultants (even though they may do little or no consulting), funds their research, and pays for the expenses of their continuing education. Equally obscured is the willingness of many doctors to accept this largesse. Trinkets bloom into meals at fine restaurants; meals grow into speaking fees; speaking fees morph into ongoing consultations and memberships on drug company advisory boards—positions that command up to six figures a year.

A massive expansion of the highly profitable drug, device, and biotechnology industries, along with the addition of large sums of money for health care has transformed medicine from a sleepy mom-and-pop operation to one of the most successful businesses in an otherwise dormant economy. Pharmaceutical companies have learned that their profits are at least as dependent on the power of their marketing efforts as the power of their scientific accomplishments, and they have pumped money into physicians' pockets in many seemingly innocuous as well as many egregious ways. This enormous infusion of money has yielded financial incentives that many physicians find difficult to ignore. In turn, these incentives yield conflicts of interest that pit the physicians' personal welfare against the welfare of their patients. They can exaggerate physicians' financial expectations, impair their judgment, create deception, inflate medical costs, erode professionalism, and harm patients. I will tell the story of physicians' everyday struggle between their professional responsibilities and their personal financial well-being.

In the middle of the twentieth century most doctors were in solo practice. Voluntary part-time faculty and a small cadre of full-time specialists populated the teaching staffs of medical centers. The principal rule governing professional behavior was the Hippocratic oath, which urged physicians in "whatever houses they visit" to "come for the benefit of the sick, remaining free of all intentional injustice, of all mischief." The financing of medical care has moved the ethical compass from that simplistic, patient-comes-first agenda to a more complex one, largely based on reimbursement for services. In the mid-1960s Medicare buttressed the fee-for-service system, which meant that physicians expected and received a fee for every visit and for most tests. But the consequent liberal spending under this payment system multiplied the cost of care, and soon insurers installed restrictive practices, hoping to control costs. Heath maintenance organizations (HMOs) became a major instrument of change. Under the HMOs, excessive charges were supplanted by restrictions of care. In fact, under both payment systems clinical practices had followed the flow of dollars. In time, as many physicians were threatened with a loss of income, they sought other sources of income. The pharmaceutical industry, and soon the biotechnology and device industries pumped huge sums into research and marketing. Much of the money was aimed at seducing practicing physicians and researchers to collaborate with the companies' marketing strategies.

Academic medicine also flourished in the 1960s, led by major growth in federal training and research programs, and the ranks of doctors in academia swelled. Threatened by Japan's industrial success and trying to copy it, Congress passed legislation that provided financial incentives for academic institutions and their researchers to patent their discoveries. Using patents from inventions of their scientists, presidents of major medical centers have eagerly tried to reap the institutional rewards of licensing agreements, but at the same time they have an abiding need to protect their faculties' pure academic pursuits. One only has to wonder what effect the exploitation of faculty ingenuity has on the kind of research the scientists engage in.

Perverse incentives do not end, however, with individual physicians. Many medical professional organizations have also become much too close to industry, and their coziness with drug companies has influenced some of their professional and lay publications. Hidden financial conflicts of interest also dog decisions made by government agencies such as the Food and Drug Administration and the National Institutes of Health, and by panels of experts in professional organizations convened to issue "clinical practice guidelines," policies that physicians use every day to diagnose and treat diseases.

Young physicians, now heavily in debt at the beginning of their careers from educational loans, are particularly vulnerable to industry's financial rewards, especially when they see their senior role models availing themselves freely of such largesse. Acceptance of lunches, dinners, and gifts from industry explains much about how idealistic medical students and house officers gradually become acculturated into accepting and later even demanding industry donations. There is a silent progression, from the innocence of accepting pens and pizza to a later winking nod that silently condones the gifts, and finally to a bland and unquestioning acceptance of pharmaceutical money by physicians as their careers advance.

The integrity of individual physicians and physician organizations is at stake. Most physicians who are close to industry swear that they are not and could not be influenced by a financial conflict of interest, yet this posture ignores what we know about human nature and the powerful influence of money. I am not naïve enough to hope for or expect moral purity in the medical profession in an imperfect world where such an attribute is a rare commodity. All gifts do not have the same impact: a pen emblazoned with the name of a company or a sandwich from a friendly pharmaceutical representative probably does not have the same influence as a well-paid seat on a company's advisory board, and any approach to reform must recognize such differences. Yet each gift is personal, and our culture is such that we tend to reciprocate in some fashion, even for small favors.

I love medicine. In my various roles as practitioner, teacher, researcher, writer, and editor, I have been thrilled to be part of an honored profession. Over more than four decades I have witnessed remarkable changes in medicine firsthand—an enormous growth in the scientific basis of medicine, an explosion of new noninvasive tests, a gratifying new armamentarium of effective new drugs, and refinements in physician-patient interactions. Thousands of physicians effectively collaborate with the pharmaceutical, biotechnology, and device industries to develop new diagnostic tools, prostheses, and medications. This book is not a criticism of these industries; others have examined their practices extensively. I am not opposed to big business, to capitalism, or to making money. Viewed from a long-term perspective, these industries have produced medications that have extended life, prevented serious illnesses, and improved the quality of life of millions of people. The companies are also a vigorous engine that accounts, in part, for our country's phenomenal economic growth. Even if we were unwilling to overlook some of the inappropriate behavior of drug, device, and biotechnology companies, we would have to conclude that overall, the companies have produced a great many products that benefit us.

In spite of this, these companies' efforts to influence physicians must give us serious pause. Many of the physicians' complex conflicts that I describe in the book are encouraged by industry, yet without the willing engagement and active involvement of physicians, many of the consequences would be lessened or eliminated. Here is the dilemma: where does the line exist between advancing the cause of science and the betterment of patient care on the one hand and the pecuniary interests of the physicians collaborating with industry to produce these advances on the other? There is little doubt that substantial sums of money induce physicians to drift across the line, and as they do, financial conflicts of interest can cause great damage.

I believe that the great majority of physicians are high-minded and principled, and that most of them intentionally avoid any kind of entanglements with industry. Their dedication to their work, their willingness to sacrifice time with their families for time at their patients' bedside, and their efforts to improve themselves and the system of care make many of them truly heroic. Nonetheless, serious conflicts of interest are widespread, and with the growth of industry marketing, they continue to increase. Whether intentionally or not, too many physicians have become marketing whores, mere tools of industry's promotional efforts. Others have engaged in pseudoscientific studies and published biased articles and educational materials that foster industry goals over patient goals. My beef is with those who exploit their professional status for personal gain in schemes that are counterproductive to patients' best interests and the profession's venerable goal of curing and caring for the sick. Clinical advice, like votes, should never be bought.

Since a warning more than 20 years ago about the threats of physician-industry involvement, enthusiasm for open discussion of the pros and cons of physicians' entanglements has never been sustained. Occasional journal articles and reports in the press, even quite recently, generate transient debates, but even reports of deaths of research subjects have a short shelf life. Nobody has wanted to raise the debate to include the entire scope of the financial arrangements between the profession and industry; there is too much money at stake. I raise it here.

Patients should not have to worry about the integrity of their doctors. They are already baffled by the choice of medical insurance, incapable of navigating the system to straighten out their medical bills, beset by increasingly expensive copayments, and dismayed about limitations in their choices of doctors and hospitals. I am reluctant to lay on still another encumbrance, yet for individual patients the consequences of their doctors' financial connections to HMOs and industry can be far reaching. Patients can be burdened by excessive and unnecessary office visits, exposed to inappropriate and dangerous diagnostic tests, given the wrong medications, forced to spend far more than necessary on prescription drugs, refused valuable tests or treatments, and exposed to potentially harmful effects in clinical research experiments. Unfortunately, they also need to know about conflict of interest.

There is little chance that financial conflicts of interest will become less prevalent or influential without active attention by the public. I am certainly not suggesting that we could or should ever return to the simple days in the middle of the last century. But the extent that financial conflicts can influence patient care and taint medical information must no longer remain hidden; to preserve the public's trust, such arrangements must become transparent. But disclosure alone is not sufficient. These associations must be shaped so that people can identify situations in which physicians' financial interests threaten patients' health and pocketbooks. Like many other societal institutions, medicine depends on the public's trust for its viability. Patients must be able to trust that their doctors' motives are not subverted by financial gain, that their doctors are recommending treatments that benefit them, and that their doctors are involving them in research projects for the right reasons. Their doctors must not only be at their sides, but on their sides.

It is time to expose the complexities and the extent of the complicity between doctors and industry. It is time to distill the benefits of these collaborations and to fully explore the risks. The combined weight of the stories I have accumulated paint a picture of members of the profession that have stepped over the boundary of appropriate behavior and caused substantial harm. Something must be done, because the health of every citizen is at stake.

ON THE TAKE

1

FREE GIFTS, FREE MEALS,
FREE EDUCATION, SPECIAL DEALS

Most physicians work hard, dedicate themselves to their patients, and preserve their professional rectitude. Tens, perhaps hundreds of thousands never take a free meal and never make a deal that could taint their clinical judgments. Unfortunately, many, often those with power and influence, have been compromised by greed. Their willingness to put personal income ahead of patients' well-being has been made possible by an enormous infusion of cash into medicine from industry, especially pharmaceutical companies. In taking meals, gifts, and trips, in joining drug company advisory boards and speaker's bureaus, and in giving industry-sponsored clinical talks and writing industry-sponsored brochures, physicians increasingly harbor financial conflicts of interest that tend to bias them in the sponsor's favor.

The very diversity of the relations is chilling; the extent of physicians' involvement is as closely guarded as clandestine military information, and nobody involved with industry wants the whole truth to be known. The full extent of the collaboration may even be undiscoverable. Nonetheless, innumerable stories about these conflicts are compelling. A sample illustrates how ubiquitous they are, who has the conflicts, and how they are manifested. These stories give a broad overview of a profession on the take.

Freebies at Medical Meetings

People outside of medicine would be dazzled to watch some physicians interact with industry representatives at medical meetings. The scene looks like a Hollywood set. Scores of beautiful men and women from pharmaceutical, biotechnology, device, and book companies greet the doctors wandering through the hall, where enormous, expensive artistic creations announce the successes of the companies' drugs with lights, sound, food, and electronic wizardry. (Dr. Jeffrey Levine, chief of psychiatry at the Bronx-Lebanon Medical Center once dubbed an annual conference of psychiatry as the "American Psychiatric Association GlaxoSmithKline Convention.")[1] At many company stations, the beautiful people hand out free stuff to any doctor who exhibits even a minimum of interest in their displays. Fifteen to twenty years ago, company representatives handed out a free packet of drug samples or a pen or pad of paper emblazoned with their company's logo. Some meetings are still like this, but at others today the stuff is better.

At many meetings, doctors congregate in clusters, making it easy to identify the exhibits at which freebies are being distributed. They look like ants congealing around drops of honey. And sometimes they are quite unruly—crowding around, pushing their way through to get a handout. At one meeting I attended, one pharmaceutical company was giving away an item the size of a thick paperback book in an unmarked white box. Even though the doctors had no idea what was being given away, they were grabbing for the boxes. At another exhibit I saw some doctors reach over and then behind one of the counters to snag a tee shirt when the drug representative couldn't get to them quickly enough. Some had shamelessly stuffed one or two shopping bags with loot. Some were lined up for a free check of their blood cholesterol.

At some meetings each of the doctors becomes a walking advertisement. At one, a cloth cord imprinted repeatedly with AstraZeneca held the nametag around the doctor's neck. At another, the nametag had two panels, one with the doctor's name and the other, below, with the company's name (Aventis Pharma) and in large letters the name of Lovenox, one of the company's new drugs that is used to prevent and treat blood clots. The convenient bags that the doctors carried at the meeting also displayed a company's logo, and inside, the meeting's program carried more advertising. Much of the loot is well marked with ads, so that the new owners of coffee mugs and tee shirts will not lose sight of their benefactors.

I attended the American Society of Nephrology meeting in 2000 and made notes as I walked through the exhibit hall. The attendees were carrying several different cloth bags advertising one drug or another, one company or another. Some bags contained only heavy programs of the meeting, others were brimming with "stuff": notepads, fans with cute cats on one side and an advertisement on the other, rubber models of red blood cells and kidneys, plastic carrots and pickles, real candy, drug samples, baseball caps, mouse pads, flashlights, and luggage tags. Doctors were standing in a long line to get postcards emblazoned with their photograph; many were standing in another line to get a personalized placard that they could hang in their office. Sponsored by Pfizer, it had their photograph in a corner and read, "What this doctor can tell you about high blood pressure can save your life." And of course there were free pens everywhere. I counted about 20 (I was too embarrassed to collect them). I thought it was interesting that no two pens were alike! Plenty of coffee, muffins, and smoothies were available; all free.

At some meetings you can't just walk up and hold out your hand to get the free stuff. Some companies require that you fill out a form containing questions about their products, and others require that you answer questions about the latest study involving one of their products. To get a free tee shirt with the drug Carvedilol on it from Roche Laboratories at one meeting, a doctor first had to answer six questions about the drug. Some questions disingenuously disguised statements about the drug's efficacy. One question asked, "Which 'C' [Carvedilol] trial is the first ever large scale study demonstrating the mortality benefit of a comprehensive adrenergic blocker in patients with severe chronic heart failure?" Another simply asked whether the attendee knew the location and time of a Roche-sponsored symposium that was being held separate from the meeting. If the doctor didn't know the answers, he or she didn't go away empty handed: someone was around to help with the answers or to correct the errors, and the second chance yielded the booty anyway.

The gifts at this meeting, of course, only seemed free. In fact, the tokens come at some personal cost to each doctor. Picking up only a pen or a notepad usually does not require that the doctor identify himself or herself, but generally the bigger gifts do. In some instances, in order to finalize a questionnaire, the doctor must supply detailed information about his practice: name, address, specialty, and type of practice. At some meetings this process is automated during the registration process by producing a magnetic card impregnated with this information. (Of course, the professional organization and the companies are in cahoots to make this possible.) The fact that the physicians have complied with the company's requirements to receive a gift also labels them as people who might be influenced by other kinds of largesse—free dinners or consulting arrangements, to name only two. Thus, in receiving a gift, the doctor has not only surrendered some of his privacy, but also identified himself as a future target for various promotions. The deals that doctors are offered are impressive.

One Doctor's Mailbox

Most people probably think that their doctor's mail is pretty much like their own: the usual bills, catalogs, credit card offers, ostensibly terrific deals from MCI, and various other solicitations. Of course, there would be some medical journals too. I doubt, however, that they know about the rest. During my eight-year tenure as editor in chief of the *New England Journal of Medicine*, physicians often sent me material that they considered a threat to the profession; some still do. In 2002, Dr. Robert E. Reisman, a senior allergist in full-time practice in Buffalo, New York sent me dozens of letters from pharmaceutical companies offering him incentives to participate in a variety of sponsored events. Some of the invitations must have been hard to turn down: a trip to Cancun, a free Palm Pilot, dinner and entertainment in fine restaurants.

Here's a close look at one month of his mail, including the payback that the companies expected. In March 2001, he received 13 invitations from major pharmaceutical companies or their surrogates.[2] The companies included AstraZeneca, Aventis, Schering, Key, Muro, Alcon, Novartis, and 3M. Five were invitations to top restaurants during the upcoming meeting of the allergy societies in New Orleans. Some offered dinner, some jazz concerts (one by Wynton Marsalis' group), the less spectacular merely "fine wines and decadent desserts." For some, guests were welcome. Attendees had no required tasks; they just had to show up.

Four of the remaining letters offered modest gifts, such as $100 gift cer-tificates. Most of these required the doctor's participation in short online or telephone surveys; one required that the physician extract information from his patients' records. One offered dinner at a local restaurant but gave no indication of what the program might entail; another offer, a kind called "dine and dash," involved meeting with a drug representative at a local restaurant while free take-out food was being prepared for his family.

The all-expense trip to Cancun included a $1,000 honorarium. It was matched by one from another company, an all-expense-paid weekend trip to the Pointe South Mountain Resort in Phoenix. The honorarium for this venture was $2,000, with an additional $100 included for incidental expenses. In exchange for attending either of these get-togethers, the physician would become capable of giving paid lectures on behalf of the company.

For some, payback involved only allowing themselves to be exposed at dinner to welcoming posters from the company, or menus emblazoned with the company's name. For others, the take-out offer for example, it required listening to the hard sell of drug reps whose knowledge is often limited to a narrow spectrum of effects and side effects of their company's newest break-through drug. The Palm Pilot offer included 1,500 frequent-flier airline miles and required that the doctor engage in online market research for the company for six months. Becoming a paid speaker for the company after a day or two training session comes with a much higher price.

In 2004, Dr. Reisman's invitations keep coming. One describes its objec-tives as "helping to build impactful marketing messages for the Zyrtec . . . franchise;"[3] another to "develop, train, and certify speakers for utilization in marketing and field-based promotional programs."[4]

While Dr. Reisman accepted none of the invitations, many doctors do.

A Surprising Quid Pro Quo

Sometimes you have no idea what to expect. In 1977, I experienced 15 minutes of fame when my colleague John Harrington and I discovered that a medication widely used by patients with high blood pressure could raise blood potassium to dangerous levels and thus cause cardiac arrest. Over the 4th of July weekend that year newspapers across the country carried headlines about our study such as "Potassium treatment questioned" (*Associated Press*), "Blood pressure RX called harmful" (*Cleveland Plain Dealer*), and "Blood pressure treatment bad for patients?" (*Miami Herald*). Within weeks I was invited to become a member of the speaker's bureau of the giant worldwide pharmaceutical company, Hoechst Roussel.

Armed with the hypothesis that a commonly prescribed diuretic, Hydrodiuril, could cause a dangerous depletion of body potassium stores, John and I spent months tracking down every relevant study of the drug and its effects. Assembling the information was far more difficult in the 1970s than now. To find studies, we had to dig through four-inch-thick, five-pound copies of the *Index Medicus*, the only compendium of published medical studies then available, using only stilted index terms under which the articles had been characterized. Over meatball subs from the local pizza parlor, we spent countless evenings away from our wives and our (in total) 11 children, assembling the data. We struggled to fit the evidence into our hypothesis, but we could not. In disbelief, we found that our hypothesis was wrong! In the medical journal *Kidney International* in June 1977, we reported that Hydrodiuril's effect on potassium was quite modest, but that the common practice of giving potassium salts to replenish potassium losses caused by Hydrodiuril could be life threatening.[5] Normal potassium levels in the blood are 4 to 5. Hydrodiuril generally reduced it to 3.5, yielding little danger, but supplementary potassium salts (the alternative to eating five or ten bananas a day) sometimes raised blood potassium to levels of 8 or 9. Such levels, we argued, could (and do) cause the heart to stop.

Somehow, the publication of this report—and maybe all the publicity—made us seem experts on diuretics and potassium metabolism. That's where Hoechst came in. Hoechst had recently introduced a new diuretic, Lasix. It was a major advance over Hydrodiuril—far more potent in extracting excessive fluid from patients with heart failure, advanced liver disease, and kidney disease, and I had prescribed it often. The Hoechst representatives offered to add me to a list of speakers that their drug representatives would offer to hospital staffs around the country. When I was chosen to speak, they would pay all of my travel expenses plus give me a $700 honorarium (about $2,000 in today's dollars). There were no strings attached. I could talk on any subject requested by the host and say whatever I wanted. In our discussions about my joining the list, neither they nor I mentioned Lasix. In fact, when I gave talks on the speaker's bureau, Hoechst's name sometimes was mentioned, but often it was not.

To this day I remember how important I felt to be chosen. I could not perceive any risk, only benefit. My reputation would be enhanced, and the $700 was a welcome addition to a rather meager fixed academic salary. The only other way of supplementing my income at the time was through speaking engagements throughout New England that paid $100 to $200, including expenses. I signed up.

For a number of years I gave several talks a year. Hoechst was true to its word. Nobody from the company suggested topics, nobody whispered in my ear to include Lasix in my talks, and there seemed to be no particular presence of Hoechst drug representatives at my talks or at my office. In fact, often the only person who knew that Hoechst sponsored me was the local director of medical education. I can't remember whether I mentioned Lasix from time to time, but I know I felt no particular compunction to do so or not to do so. After several years on the speaker's bureau, a Hoechst representative offered to send me to a public relations firm on Madison Avenue in New York for training in public speaking. The experience, he said, could groom me for possible video appearances. After a rather glamorous, ego-building encounter with these professionals, the representatives said that I was ready for bigger things, including trips to bigger places. Participation in this new program had only one requirement. I had to mention Lasix at least once in each of my talks.

I refused. I felt uncomfortable with what seemed like a questionable practice. My invitations to speak for Hoechst abruptly ended.

Gifts and Fees

Interactions between pharmaceutical companies and physicians often begin with visits from drug reps (so-called detail men and women). These visits are frequent, and often these salesmen (who now number 87,000) aggressively promote their newest drugs while bearing gifts and lunches.[6] The reps visit practicing doctors in their offices and are seen all over hospitals and academic medical centers, often bearing yet more gifts. Over the years physicians have received gifts of all kinds including meals at the best restaurants, tickets to sporting events, invitations to resorts with spouses included, breakfasts and lunches for their office staff or trainees, and cash payments. As in the past, some physicians accept free samples on an ongoing basis from pharmaceutical representatives. Rather than use them for their indigent patients, they take them for themselves and their family members even though they certainly can afford to buy the drugs themselves.

Some physicians became paid consultants to drug and biotechnology companies. Though some serve on scientific committees that deal with aspects of drug development, others sit on internal committees and boards of directors and become engaged in the business aspects (including marketing) of the companies. Some of these physicians have influence over the drugs that their hospitals and organizations use every day. Others consult for the investment industry (Morgan Stanley, for example), and the food industry. Many have joined the speaker's bureau of one company or many companies, and are paid for lecturing in a medical domain vital to the company's marketing interests.

Medical professional organizations such as the American Thoracic Society, the Society for Critical Care Medicine, and the Endocrine Society are also deeply involved with industry, and many receive large payments that they use to support scientific meetings, professional education, and ongoing operating expenses. In some instances pharmaceutical and other companies offer inducements without prompting, but often leaders of the organization solicit funding from industry, sometimes for specific programs. Companies frequently offer funds for a medical society's awards given out at annual meetings of these societies. The awards often have joint names: the organization's and the company's (for example, the Eli Lilly and Company Research Award of the American Society of Microbiology, the ACC (American College of Cardiology) Merck Cardiology Fellowship Awards, the APIRE (the research foundation of the American Psychiatric Association)/GlaxoSmithKline Award). Some are highly prestigious, and some come with large cash prizes that accrue to the honored individual. Some companies fund professorships and contribute to the endowment of medical schools. Virtually all sponsor research at academic medical centers, and the amount spent in these institutions is enormous. Many medical centers could not get along without the large overhead payments that accompany such grants.

The drug industry spent approximately two billion dollars in 2001 alone for meetings and events for physicians, a figure that represents a doubling over the past five years.[7] Speakers, funded by one company or another, are brought in at major medical centers to offer continuing education programs. At some, virtually all the speakers invited to speak to the staff in a division (cardiology, for example) or a department (psychiatry, for example) are sponsored by industry. The companies heavily subsidize lectures for physicians in all kinds of locations: hospitals, local hotels and restaurants, at medical meetings, in free-standing conferences, in video conference facilities. The estimated cost of these education activities in 1999 was more than half a billion dollars. It goes without saying that the companies aren't doing this purely for altruistic reasons.[8] Pharmaceutical companies have myriad other ways of subsidizing physicians. They pay physicians in practice $2,000 to $4,000 for enrolling individual patients into drug trials, and offer additional bonuses of $2,000 to $3,000 when enrollment slows down over the holiday season.[9] It is not difficult for a busy physician to bring in tens of thousands of dollars a year from such patient enrollments.

In recent years, the pharmaceutical industry's aggressive marketing efforts have come to public attention. Some of the extraordinary subsidies that physicians have taken have been revealed, and the complex conflicts of interest that gifts and subsidies generate have been exposed. In response, some organizations have introduced new guidelines about industry-physician interactions. The American Medical Association (AMA) allows physicians to take gifts if they entail a benefit to patients and only if they are not of "substantial value," and meals if they are "modest" ones.[10] Thus, pens, notepads, office items, and books are still considered acceptable, but tickets to sporting events and dinners that often include spouses (both previously ubiquitous) are not. In mid-2002, PhRMA, the Pharmaceutical Manufacturers Association, issued its own guidelines that are similar to those of the AMA.[11]

Implied in the PhRMA guidelines is an intention to cut back on money spent on physicians, but I have my doubts. Gifts and subsidies are so important to the marketing efforts of industry that the companies will undoubtedly find creative ways to continue the largesse. Given the extraordinary competition between companies for sales of their new products, even if effective restrictions are placed on expenditures for physicians, it is quite likely that the companies will greatly increase the money they spend on physicians for consulting, on medical journal advertising, and on advertising directly to consumers. Where the marketing balloon deflates in one sector, it will undoubtedly inflate in another. Such is the lure and power of marketing.

The Allure of Meals

Food is an extremely important sales tool, and there is little limit to the meals that physicians receive from drug companies. In most academic medical centers, community hospitals, and Veterans Administration hospitals, house staff conferences and specialty conferences are held in the early morning and at noon, and drug salesmen frequently bring in the meals. They hand out brochures and engage the participants in conversation about their latest products. Sometimes the salesmen are allowed to give a 15 to 20 minute presentation. Heads of departments often solicit the meals from representatives of several companies.

Though the meals brought into hospitals for trainees usually fit the AMA's "modest" criterion (pasta, pizza, or sandwiches), outside the institutions dinner meetings are usually held at upscale restaurants. Already, less than a year after the PhRMA guidelines were issued, there is evidence that the companies are violating their own guidelines on meals, and despite the new AMA guidelines, physicians are still accepting their invitations. An analysis of restaurants in the Philadelphia area where industry-sponsored meals were held showed that on average, the pharmaceutical dinners were about 40 percent more expensive than the average in the Zagat restaurant guide.[12] Pharmaceutical dinners in 2004 in Buffalo and New Haven still include the most expensive restaurants. The price of a ticket to these restaurant dinners is to listen to the salesman in what is generally described as an "educational discussion," though such talks often end up in conversations about a single drug manufactured by the sponsoring company.

Physicians in the community, especially "big prescribers" of drugs, are also generously treated to meals, and they also sometimes solicit the meals (which are shared by their office staff) in exchange for an encounter with the pharmaceutical salesman. Chris Adams described particularly flagrant examples of exploitation in the *Wall Street Journal*. He reported that Dr. Charles Field, an internal medicine specialist in New Orleans, had participated in a "dine and dash" event at Martin Wine Cellar. The invitation for the event (labeled, "Why Cook?"), read, "Come in and order dinner for you and your family." More than a dozen physicians likely to prescribe drugs for arthritis gathered to meet representatives of Merck and Co. for wine and deli sandwiches. Merck, with its new Cox-2 inhibitor, Vioxx, (an expensive one-pill-a-day treatment for arthritis) was then engaged in a head-to-head competition with Pfizer over Pfizer's Cox-2 inhibitor, Celebrex. In the interview with Adams, Dr. Field bragged that he sometimes participated in these events twice in one day, that he had gone to such events as often as five times in one week, that he had accepted two Christmas trees courtesy of a company, and that he estimated that he had attended 150 to 200 such events in the course of two years. One time, he said, he attended three events, a dinner, a dine and dash, and a trip to a local bookstore for a free book in one day. Dr. Field admitted that dinners and gifts do influence the drugs he prescribes, but he claimed they do only in marginal situations, when he believes that two drugs are equivalent in their effectiveness. Dr. John Ernst, another New Orleans doctor who often accepts dinner invitations, offered the common excuse that he and his wife (who doesn't like to cook) would go out for dinner anyway. He is convinced that his associations with industry are valuable, but not, he said, "from the profiteering I get from the free dinner, which obviously I don't need."[13] Dine and dash events are no longer permitted under the PhRMA code, but invitations to meals at expensive restaurants still arrive.

Making Friends When They're Young

Interns and residents, a young, underappreciated, hard-working, and debt-ridden group, often develop a kind of siege mentality focused around the stress of their demanding schedules, which has them working 80-hour weeks and as many as 30 hours straight. Within this mind-set they are susceptible to a narrow set of desires: more sleep, more encouragement, a few hours of relaxation, a little kindness, and free, accessible food. Drug company representatives appreciate these vulnerabilities and needs, and step in to help. I witnessed a typical lunch that was sponsored by Pfizer at an academic medical center.[14] Two well-dressed pharmaceutical representatives in their late 20s or early 30s had brought food from the outside for a regular teaching conference (which I was giving) for the house staff in an academic medical center. One by one, house officers and medical students arrived to join a buffet line and were greeted warmly by the male drug rep with "How was your weekend?" or "How're you doing?" These reps were obviously a familiar presence. The line moved slowly because it took some time to scoop up the salad, the pasta, and the chicken marsala onto paper plates. The two drug reps used this opportunity to make a pitch for the company's products. One was stationed strategically at the beginning of the line, and the other at the end. I was nearly out of earshot, but I heard the reps describe two of the company's popular products as well as recommendations for dosages. Many of the attendees in the line seemed to be listening less out of interest in the sales pitch than out of courtesy toward those who had spared them the expense and bother of getting fed. The female drug rep, at the end of the line, seemed particularly to engage the male house officers. Lunch isn't the end of it. On one evening in a pizza joint in New Haven, I observed a resident in scrubs with his team of interns and students enjoying pizza and beer with a drug representative. There were two "costs" for the free food and drinks. The resident had to listen to the drug rep's sales pitch during the meal, and at the end of the party he was given a pile of reprints to take back to the rest of his team.

One evening during dinner at one of the best restaurants in a university town with the chief residents of a major academic medical center (I was their visiting professor for two days), I watched with amusement as my guests waved to many of their colleagues as they filed into the back room to have dinner and receive a free textbook from a drug company salesman. I was amused because at that particular medical center the chairman of their department had made a powerful ethical statement by subsidizing all of the meals that house officers receive during conferences from departmental funds; no drug company money was accepted. The lesson had been lost on many.

Nonwork by Well-Paid Consultants

It might be useful to coin the term "pseudoconsultant," to refer to those physicians invited to restaurants or resorts to consult for a company, but being asked to consult on little more than which wine to order. This practice was revealed in the global settlement for fraud between various governmental parties and TAP Pharmaceuticals, Inc. over inappropriate marketing and sales of the drug Lupron. The report of the settlement describes all-expenses-paid weekends at resorts that included such important consulting activities as golf, skiing, and white-water rafting.[15] It says: "The doctors were in fact not typical consultants; indeed few of the normal trappings of consultancy existed: no consultant reports were prepared; the doctors never billed TAP for their time; . . . And the sales employees who nominated the doctors to attend the 'consulting' programs typically had no discussions with the doctors regarding the consulting services to be provided or that 'had been provided' during the course of the weekend event. . . . . [This supports] the conclusion that in fact the physicians were not consultants and were merely receiving a benefit from TAP in their attendance at the event."

In-Kind Substitutes for Payments

If pharmaceutical companies are constrained in giving gifts, educational grants, free trips, and expensive meals, what will they substitute in their attempts to ingratiate themselves with physicians, especially those in leadership positions? As mentioned before, loopholes allow them to make physicians consultants to their companies, but because the practice of pseudoconsulting has already come under fire, they will undoubtedly turn to other tactics. In one such approach, a company offered free administrative consulting services to help a group of physicians better manage their offices.[16] The same kinds of arrangements are occurring in academic medical centers. One physician, who asked not to be named, forwarded to me an e-mail in which a drug salesman offered to bring her business partner to meet with the head of the hospital's intensive care unit on topics such as reimbursement for services, quality measures, clinical outcomes, and patient flow.[17]

A Piece of the Action

More and more researchers, including those involved in clinical research, are working hand-in-hand with companies to develop new drugs and devices, encouraged by federal legislation intended to enhance the country's productivity and competitiveness. In the course of these activities, investigators are becoming part owners of patents and small companies, and some have received stock or stock options in companies worth hundreds of thousands of dollars. These arrangements become conflicts of interest when the researchers use their own inventions and discoveries on their own patients, when they promote the new drugs and devices, especially when they do not disclose that they might profit from the use of the new materials, or when they devote their time to these profit-making activities and ignore their university responsibilities.

Subsidized Education

If a practicing doctor plays his cards right, he may not have to pay to keep up to date with modern advances in medicine. An enormous amount of continuing medical education (CME) is subsidized by industry. Before 1940, most of the medical schools had a few continuing education courses for practicing physicians, but attendance was low. At that time, once doctors passed a certifying examination (by the American Board of Internal Medicine or the American Board of Surgery, for example) they remained certified for life. Rapid advances in the pharmaceutical industry after the Second World War changed all of this. Many drugs were introduced for the treatment of high blood pressure, edema (swelling), infections, and diseases of the immune system. New methods of imaging inner organs also began to emerge. These advances were soon followed by an extraordinary proliferation of new drugs to treat certain cancers, to lower blood cholesterol, and to manage psychiatric conditions and glandular disorders. Human organ transplantation became a reality and new noninvasive therapeutic techniques were introduced.

Over the years these remarkable changes in medical practice generated a new need for physicians in practice to "keep up." Nonetheless, AMA members objected to mandatory requirements and as a result, participation in continuing medical education remained voluntary. Where the AMA faltered, however, many state medical societies stepped in and required CME by mandating attendance at courses as a prerequisite for membership and licensure.[18] Initially, academic medical centers and medical schools expanded their offerings to meet the growing demand. Physicians paid a modest fee, attended the lectures, and received "Category 1 credits" that they counted toward the education requirements of state boards or state medical societies. A few academic departments actually found that setting up such courses could be quite profitable.

Unfortunately, there were many abuses as industry became involved. Physicians often attended meetings that were held in resorts, foreign countries, and on cruise ships. In some instances, they could sign in as having attended the meeting, get credit for attendance, but go off to see the sights or play golf. Some directors of CME programs, eager to encourage participants to keep coming to their meetings, looked the other way at such infractions. At some meetings, for example, the sign-up for credits was on the honor system. Physicians would sign up in the morning, go out to play golf or tennis, and then sign in later for full credit.

During the 1970s and 1980s, pharmaceutical companies occasionally offered financial support for such programs in the form of unrestricted grants in exchange for recognition of such sponsorship, but the companies rarely tried to influence the content of the programs and were content to leave the choice of programs and faculty to the organizers. As late as 1986, few commercial organizations were offering CME, but for-profit organizations known as "medical education and communication companies," and "medical education service suppliers" soon appreciated that medical centers weren't the only ones that could put on educational programs for doctors. Moreover, the pharmaceutical and device industries were quite willing to support the efforts of these commercial organizations in return for the marketing opportunities they offered. The medical education companies could not do the teaching, of course, because they did not have the professional expertise, but they quickly appreciated that they could hire academic physicians and community "thought leaders" (also known as "key opinion leaders") not only to do the teaching for them but also develop the programs and hire the faculty for the courses. Lobbying efforts and threats of legal action by these commercial education companies ultimately led the Accreditation Council for Continuing Education (ACCME), the independent body that accredits educational organizations, to give accreditation authority to the commercial education providers, and the flood gates for commercialization of CME were opened.[19] The hegemony of academia over CME ended abruptly, at a time when support for medical education by hospitals and universities was already in decline. Once the drug companies began subsidizing the commercial suppliers, much continuing medical education became free.

More than 100 for-profit entities are accredited now, including medical education and communication companies, medical education service suppliers, publishing companies such as Lippincott Williams and Wilkins and Excerpta Medica, several insurance companies, a managed-care trade group, an auction company, and at least one pharmaceutical company (Eli Lilly), to provide highly sophisticated CME to America's doctors.[20] CME has become a major commercial enterprise. According to Public Citizen, a watchdog organization in Washington, DC, a survey by a medical marketing company estimated that in 1999 the yearly revenues for commercial CME suppliers was more than 600 million dollars, and it is still growing.[21] About three-quarters of the income of these commercial companies is derived from pharmaceutical companies.

On the local level, drug companies (or their surrogates in the medical education business) frequently sponsor conferences in hospitals or in local restaurants and hotels. Often, specialists from institutions outside the city are brought in, presumably because they deliver messages consistent with the company's marketing missions. At meetings of specialty organizations, such as the American Heart Association, the American Society of Nephrology, and the American Gastroenterological Association, many industry-sponsored talks are held outside the scientific program. The official program usually begins at 8:00 AM and finishes at 5:00 or 6:00 PM, but before the official program begins and after it ends, pharmaceutical-company-sponsored "symposia" offer exposure to important academic speakers accompanied by breakfast or dinner. The specialty society approves these "satellite" symposia, receives some payment for allowing them, and allows its mailing list to be used ahead of time to mail glossy brochures created by the pharmaceutical companies' agents announcing time, place, and subject matter. Very often university departments of continuing medical education provide education credits to the doctors who attend the symposia. These departments collect a fee for developing the program and issuing the CME credits.

At the 2002 American Heart Association meeting, for example, there were 30 "free" symposia sponsored by one drug (or device) company or another.[22] Many of the speakers had financial arrangements with the companies sponsoring the meeting. The professional organization typically has no say in the content of the program or the choice of speakers, but the society is rewarded for allowing companies to put on the programs. In fact, while all the hoopla is going on at the medical meetings, and while some doctors are collecting shopping bags full of pens and pads, some academic physicians are fattening their bank accounts by teaching at these pharmaceutical-company-sponsored "symposia." In 2001 one prominent medical specialist from Boston gave four lectures at different hotels the day before the American Heart Association meeting and one more at 8:00 PM on a day of the meeting. Four different pharmaceutical companies supported the five lectures, and this particular academician, who honestly (I assume) listed his conflicts of interest, was a consultant for all four companies and is on the speaker's bureau for four of them. To top it off, in one of the 2001 symposia, he gave a short, impassioned talk about the merits of the company that sponsored the event. Were his talks biased? Even if they were, I'm not sure that many could tell, but the listeners could easily take away from his lecture the need to use the newest, probably the most expensive drug, and possibly even one that might not be as effective as the one that they are accustomed to using.

How much the meeting coordinators and speakers get paid for doing this is a closely guarded secret, but another prominent cardiologist bragged to a young colleague that he made more than $100,000 at a single meeting of the American Heart Association for these "extracurricular" activities. To do so, he had a car waiting for him as he dashed, presumably breathlessly, from one hotel to another to make the necessary appearances. No doubt he's not the only one who does this. But he's a prominent figure, and maybe he's worth it.

The claim, often heard by those who offer CME programs that they would be unable to provide these programs without industry support is untested. Clearly, without industry support there would be fewer CME programs—or fewer programs of certain types, and less lavish food, drinks, and entertainment—but that doesn't mean that there would not be sufficient programs to meet legitimate CME needs. It is even possible that by eliminating the biases created by industry support, the remaining programs would be even more valuable.

How Widespread Are the "Deals"?

Highly reliable information on financial conflicts of interest among practicing physicians and medical researchers is difficult to obtain. Surveys generally find that the research of approximately one-quarter of academic researchers is funded at least in part by industry. In a revealing survey, more than 40 percent of "life-science" researchers at 50 universities had accepted gifts of research equipment and materials, discretionary funds, trips to meetings, and a large majority of these researchers believed that the gifts were important to carrying out their work. Senior faculty received far more gifts than junior faculty: the percent of full professors, associate professors, assistant professors, and others who received gifts lined up as follows: 48 percent, 41 percent, 38 percent, and 29 percent.[23] The fact that about half of the senior academics had received gifts seemed in keeping with my hunch, based on observations from other sources, that companies focused their largesse more on the most influential people, namely those with the highest academic rank. Even these figures may underestimate the extent of industry involvement in clinical research.

Little is known about the changing extent of faculty involvement with industry. One study, however, tracked financial disclosures over a 19-year period, ending in 1999, at a single academic institution. Among 225 researchers there were 488 disclosures in the period. The disclosures increased over time, but especially over the last six years of the study.[24]

The extent of the involvement between academics and industry is well hidden, but sources close to the pharmaceutical industry inadvertently spilled the beans. The Washington Legal Foundation (WLF) is an organization devoted in part to protecting the pharmaceutical industry from excessive regulation by the FDA and the ACCME. Through lobbying efforts and court challenges, the WLF tries to insure that physicians with financial ties to industry are not prevented from participating in these education programs. In January 2003, when the ACCME tried again to exclude anyone with a financial conflict of interest from involvement in physicians' educational activities, the WLF countered aggressively on the grounds that ACCME could not prove that education by conflicted educators was biased in favor of the companies that pay them.[25] To further defend their stance, they claimed that physicians' education would suffer if those with financial conflicts were excluded from teaching. In making this point they admitted: "It is widely acknowledged that most of the top medical authorities in this country, and virtually all of the top speakers on medical topics, are employed in some capacity by one or more of the country's pharmaceutical companies. That is how it should be." They went on, "Indeed, it is difficult to understand how the [ACCME] Task Force believes that CME providers will be able to locate speakers knowledgeable regarding the latest compounds in development—except among those medical professionals being compensated by the company that is financing the development."

Given the close relation between this foundation and the pharmaceutical industry, their statement concerning the extent of financial ties between leaders in medicine and industry must be viewed as authoritative.

If the conflicts of interest listed in the program book for the Society of American Gastrointestinal Endoscopic Surgeons (SAGES) 2003 Conference is any indication of the extent of such conflicts among surgeons, they, too, are extensive. For this meeting, voluntary disclosures of financial relationships with companies ranged from research grants, serving on the company's speakers' bureau, consulting, or holding stock options. Sixty percent of the senior surgeons (professors or chiefs of departments) and 40 percent of junior surgeons (assistant professors) had at least one financial conflict. The average number of conflicts per surgeon was approximately two, though two individuals had ties with five companies. The junior surgeons with financial conflicts were generally from high-profile medical institutions (Duke, UCSF, Tufts, and Emory).[26] Even though the information is incomplete, many senior leaders in academic clinical medicine have financial conflicts of interest that could influence their research, opinions, and writing.

The secrecy surrounding financial conflicts and the reluctance to disclose the conflicts is impressive. Drug companies do not provide public lists of the physicians on their speaker's bureaus or advisory boards, and physician groups, hospitals, and academic medical centers may have lists in their files, but the information is not available in public documents. In fact, even in medical centers that have had disclosure rules about financial conflicts for some time, many chairs of departments look the other way in the hope that their faculty members will make enough income from their "outside" activities to stop bothering them about their departmental compensation. (One chairman of a Department of Medicine told me quite confidently that nobody in his department was making more than $10,000 a year in outside income. Yet only weeks earlier one of his midlevel staff members who had given a drug company talk in the exhibit hall of a major medical meeting admitted to me that he had brought in six figures in one year in personal income from the company that sponsored the exhibit.)[27]

Nonetheless, the secrecy is not absolute, and with persistent investigative effort, some information on the financial conflicts of individuals can be found, though the sources of information provide no data about dollar amounts. For several years, participants in courses or lectures accredited by the ACCME have been required to disclose their financial conflicts to the participating physicians. (Unfortunately, this requirement is often practiced in the breach. Often the printed material handed out in conjunction with the course contains no mention of the conflict, and instead, at the start of the talk, the lecturer quickly flashes a slide or two [or three] with the names of the companies with which he has a financial relationship. You have to be a speed-reader and have a photographic memory to catch more than a name or two.) The ACCME disclosure requirement, however, does create a vast source of information on financial conflicts of participants in CME programs. As examples, a teaching program in infectious diseases (NISE) and in another on gastrointestinal conditions (the 5th International Symposium on Functional Gastrointestinal Disorders) reveal extensive financial involvement of the faculty with sponsoring companies. The American Heart Association requires disclosure of the conflicts of interest of participants in company-sponsored symposia at their major annual meeting. These disclosures also reveal that senior clinical researchers are heavily involved with industry. Most have research funding and many are paid consultants, on advisory boards, and on speakers' bureaus.

Many medical journals such as the *Journal of the American Medical Association* (*JAMA*) and the *New England Journal of Medicine* require authors of scientific articles to declare their financial associations (including consulting fees, service on advisory boards, ownership of equity, patent royalties, honorariums for lectures, fees for expert testimony, and research grants), and the journals often (but not invariably) publish these associations along with the article. I began to sense the extent of involvement of academics with industry during my tenure as editor in chief of the *New England Journal of Medicine*. During that time our policy only allowed physicians (mostly academic physicians) to write review articles (papers that summarized a field) and editorials if they were free of financial conflicts with any company whose products (or their competitors) were featured in the article.[28] To insure that there were no such arrangements, we required that potential authors disclose all of their industry connections before we could give them the go-ahead to write the article. Finding authors without such conflicts seemed to get progressively more difficult during the 1990s. By the end of the 1990s we occasionally had to reject five or six prominent potential authors before we found one who had no conflicts. Indeed, my successor as editor, Dr. Jeffrey Drazen, changed the policy in 2002. He had basic disagreements with it, and in justifying the change he explained that he found it extremely difficult to find authors who were free of conflicts.[29]

Publications of clinical research give us additional hints. A *New England Journal of Medicine* article in 2002 on the antidepression drug, nefazodone, lists 29 authors. The editor's note stated: "Readers should know—that all but 1 . . . of the 12 principal authors have had financial associations with Bristol-Myers Squibb—which also sponsored the study—and, in most cases, with many other companies producing psychoactive pharmaceutical agents. The associations include consultancies, receipt of research grants and honorariums, and participation on advisory boards. Of the 17 other authors, 2 are employees of Bristol-Myers Squibb, 5 . . . have no relevant additional financial ties, and the others have a variety of associations similar to those just mentioned."[30]

Even more revealing was the admission by the editors that the conflicts were so extensive that they were unwilling to use valuable space in the paper pages of the journal to print them, so they published them instead on the *Journal*'s Web site. Printed out, the authors' financial conflicts encompassed three single-spaced typewritten pages!

Articles in *JAMA* describing "consensus conferences" (summaries of a conference devoted to a medical subject) are also revealing. The disclosure statements for one such conference on obesity in 1996 and another on AIDS in 2000 revealed that almost all of the conference participants (they had become authors) had financial conflicts and many had arrangements with several companies.[31]

Brochures edited and written by prestigious physicians and sponsored by industry also reveal complex conflicts. The authors of some, such as *Lipid Letter*, Lipids Online, and *Lipid Management*, all publications that promote statin drug use for high blood cholesterol (and are all supported by statin manufacturers) have financial ties with virtually all the companies that make statins. The *Lipid Letter* for December 2002 provides an example of how extensive financial arrangements can be: The eight physicians responsible for this Pfizer-sponsored newsletter listed that they were consulting (or were members of the speaker's bureau) for an average of six separate pharmaceutical companies. One person listed nine, and one listed 16! All eight had financial relations with the company that sponsored the brochure.[32] Many more of these industry-sponsored organizations exist.

All of these sources paint a picture of extensive involvement between academic medicine and industry, and give credence to the Washington Legal Foundation's assertion that a large fraction of the leaders in medical centers are receiving money from industry.

Additional information is available on involvement of the country's leading researchers who advise the Food and Drug Administration (FDA), and these revelations are especially disturbing because the FDA is responsible for deciding which drugs get approved for use by physicians. Dennis Cauchon, in *USA Today*, noted that from 1998 to 2000, the FDA waived federal restrictions on conflict of interest numerous times to allow experts to testify about drugs in the FDA's 18 advisory committees. He found that at 88 of 159 advisory committee meetings, half or more of the committee members had financial interests in the topic being evaluated. Of the 102 meetings that involved specific drugs, Cauchon learned that one-third of the committee members had a direct financial stake in the outcome.[33] In some instances these relationships might have endangered the health of the public.[34]

Government policies about conflict of interest are very stringent; that is, they are supposed to be. In 1994, when I was at the *New England Journal of Medicine*, I invited Dr. Harold Varmus, then the NIH director, to give the prestigious Shattuck Lecture in Boston and to have dinner at my house with a group of academic medical leaders. Varmus agreed to give the lecture, but declined the dinner invitation, explaining that the NIH conflict of interest regulations precluded him from accepting anything more than minimal meals. I had assumed that as Varmus did, all other scientists at the NIH had followed the strictest interpretation of the conflict-of-interest rules. Given this inclination, I was greatly surprised at David Willman's expose in the *Los Angeles Times* about major conflicts of interest among some of the most prestigious scientists at the NIH. In an investigation that took five years, Willman discovered that in 1995 Varmus had quietly rescinded the policy that barred institute directors from accepting consulting fees and payments of stock from companies. Thereafter scientists could develop financial relations with industry as long as they received permission from their supervisors; permission was generally given. In addition, most of the financial arrangements were kept secret.[35]

Willman discovered not only that some scientists had lucrative financial arrangements, receiving up to $600,000 over a ten-year period, but also that some were in a decision-making role that could affect the company's welfare, a direct conflict of interest. He found, for example, that Dr. Stephen Katz, director of the National Institute of Arthritis and Musculoskeletal Diseases, had collected $140,000 from Advanced Tissue Sciences, which itself had received $1.5 million in grants from Katz's institute before going bankrupt. Willman reported that Dr. Thomas Kindt, director of research at the National Institute of Allergy and Infectious Diseases had been paid $63,000 in consulting fees by Innovir Laboratories and was named an inventor on one of Innovir's patents. Willman also reported that Dr. Ronald Germain, deputy director of the NIH's Laboratory of Immunology, had taken fees "from a company collaborating formally with his laboratory." Several of the top NIH scientists had consulted with a number of outside companies. In each instance, the scientists had received permission from their supervisors. Many had received permission from Dr. Ruth Kirschstein, then acting director of the NIH. When these revelations were published, Dr. Kirschstein opined that none of the arrangements had compromised the public interest because NIH scientists and directors are "highly ethical people with enormous integrity."[36] The current NIH director, Dr. Elias Zerhouni, agreed, and said that he had found no evidence that "medical decisions had been influenced by company payments to agency officials."[37]

Nonetheless, members of Congress have demanded a full investigation, and Dr. Zerhouni, promised a thorough one. He advised NIH managers to "use prudence in accepting outside compensation,"[38] and in a memo, he said, "Please consider the greater good of the NIH when deciding whether to accept financial benefits offered in recognition of your work or public service."[39] He later reported that the NIH's top scientists were no longer accepting consulting fees or stock options, and said, "My viewpoint is very simple." There should be "a separation of oversight and management. You can't have individuals that have a direct fiduciary relationship also having a conflicting relationship."[40]

The Center for Science in the Public Interest, a not-for-profit group dedicated to ethical scientific behavior, maintains a searchable database on financial conflict of interests of American physicians, including many physicians identified from sources such as journal and educational disclosure statements.[41] However, many physicians with major conflicts are not represented on the site. Taken together, all these sources are not sufficiently complete to identify whether a given individual has a financial conflict with a company about whose drug he has spoken or written. Moreover, the extent of the financial involvement with industry is almost never disclosed. Such information often sits in the archives of medical schools and academic medical centers and never sees the light of day.

The picture that emerges here is a profession that blithely accepts gifts, dinners, trips, phony consulting arrangements, and free continuing education. Even though the extent of physician involvement with industry is not made public, evidence suggests that a great many are collaborating, and that many have financial deals with multiple companies.

MONEY-WARPED BEHAVIOR

W<small>E HAVE NOW ESTABLISHED THAT FINAN-</small>cial conflicts of interest are rife in medicine. In fact, conflicting responsibilities are a commonplace characteristic of everyday life, in politics, and in business. So why be so concerned about doctors' conflicts? The numerous examples in this chapter all lead to the same results: risk or injury to patients, flaws in medical information, and serious ethical lapses.

"If You've Got the Money, . . . I've Got the Time"[1]

Some physicians become known as whores. Whore is a strong descriptor, but I heard it repeatedly from colleagues about physicians who tour the country for drug companies, changing their talks repeatedly to hawk the products of the company that is sponsoring their visits. Still, I held back using the "W" word until the wife of a prominent academic physician in a major medical center used it to describe her husband. I asked the woman (a good and longtime friend) if she could give me some "inside information" about how often her husband (Dr. Omega, I'll call him) went out on the lecture circuit and a rough idea of how much money he brought home for these lectures. Initially she offered the information that Dr. Omega often was out one or two nights a week, and that when expenses mounted for college tuitions, he could be away for as much as two weeks at a time. She said that even though various companies pay him, he never promoted any specific product. When I began to ask about dollar amounts, my friend became anxious, blurted out that she "couldn't do this" because my book would "ruin her lifestyle," and I promptly stopped asking further questions. However, I later learned that Mrs. Omega's description of her husband was accurate. When I asked a colleague at another medical center to name some physicians who clearly had promoted certain products at lectures that he had heard in the past year, one physician he mentioned immediately without prompting was Dr. Omega. He said it was obvious that Dr. Omega had not only been pushing one particular medication over others, but did not disclose that his lecture fees and travel expenses had been sponsored by the company that sells Dr. Omega's favored drug. There are many Dr. Omegas. How many, I do not know.

Speaker's Bureaus

Pharmaceutical, biotechnology, and device companies recruit physicians (usually high-placed academic physicians and well-respected community leaders) to be members of company-supported speakers panels. These lists are circulated to hospitals and physician groups across the country, which select speakers for their various educational programs. The sponsoring companies pay speakers' expenses and provide an honorarium, usually not less than $1,000 and (depending on the prestige of the speaker) often considerably more.

There are dangers in signing on to be a speaker sponsored by a pharmaceutical company. One danger is the obligation of reciprocity, which can subconsciously (or consciously) influence a physician to become a marketing agent for the sponsor. Another way physicians might be influenced is by the subtle pressure that comes from the knowledge that they might be removed from the speakers' list if they fail to promote the sponsor's products. There is also little doubt that some speakers "hold back" from criticizing companies' products when the company is buying the butter for their bread.

At the extreme are instances in which physicians knowingly become spokespersons for the marketing efforts of a company without disclosing it. Appointment to the speaker's bureau is sometimes used as "payback" for participation in clinical drug trials. This is a ploy used to allow the trial participants to claim, honestly, that they had no financial conflict during the time that they are involved in the trial.

It is difficult to estimate the number of physicians who participate in speaker's bureaus. There probably are thousands, but speaker's bureau lists are not public documents. Given that there are new constraints on some kinds of pharmaceutical promotions, chances are that speaker's bureaus will be expanding. Such an expansion depends, of course, on physicians' willingness to participate.

Blatant Promotion of Off-Label Drugs

Another example of physicians involved with marketing is the advertising of "off-label" drugs. An off-label use of a drug is the prescribing by a doctor of a drug that has been approved by the Food and Drug Administration (FDA) for one particular condition, but the prescription is being used for a condition for which the drug has not been approved. Although it is entirely legal for a doctor to use a drug off-label, it is illegal for a drug company to advertise a drug for any purpose other than the one or ones approved by the FDA. By recruiting physicians to discuss off-label uses, therefore, the drug companies, in essence, bypass official channels and create a potent marketing force of physicians. One flagrant example of physicians aiding in marketing came to light when a whistleblower charged that Warner-Lambert (now a branch of Pfizer) had engaged in unlawful off-label marketing of the anti-epilepsy drug, Neurontin. In May 2004, Pfizer pled guilty to Medicaid fraud and agreed to pay fines of approximately $430 million.[2]

Melody Petersen, a reporter at the *New York Times*, who tracked the Neurontin story from the beginning, reported that several physicians had been paid large sums to speak about "more than a dozen other medical uses that were not approved by the Food and Drug Administration."[3] Doctors were paid to give lectures about the use of Neurontin for pain and psychiatric disorders, with the content of their talks approved by the pharmaceutical company through an intermediate. Some speakers were paid tens of thousands of dollars annually to recommend off-label uses of the drug. Doctors were also paid as "consultants" to the company when they did no consulting, but instead came to meetings where unapproved uses of the drug were touted. Doctors received tens of thousands of dollars to "act as a surrogate sales force for the company" and to prescribe the drug. The heavy subscribers were encouraged to apply to the drug company for cash payments euphemistically called "educational grants." According to Ms. Petersen's report, one, Dr. B. J. Wilder, formerly a professor at the University of Florida, received more than $300,000 over a three-year period. She also reported that a Harvard professor, Dr. Steven Schachter, received more than $70,000, and a University of Minnesota professor, Dr. Ilo Leppik, received nearly $50,000.

Medical publications also market off-label drugs. Provigil is a new drug produced by Cephalon, Inc. that increases wakefulness; its action is similar to other stimulants such as amphetamines. At the present time the FDA has approved it for use in narcolepsy, an uncommon condition in which sufferers have an overwhelming feeling of sleepiness. A 2003 supplement of *The Primary Care Companion to the Journal of Clinical Psychiatry* contains several articles about medical conditions characterized by fatigue such as depression, as well as a new entity called "executive dysfunction" in which people have a tendency to be less awake than someone thinks they should be. "Executive dysfunction" is supposedly characterized by fatigue, forgetfulness, apathy, bad mood, and inability to communicate clearly. It is said to have "no standard medical definition" and is better regarded as a "concept."[4] Although each article in the supplement contains a disclaimer that Provigil is not approved for these conditions, virtually the entire issue is a thinly disguised pitch to use Provigil for them. Cephalon paid for a teleconference at which the material in the supplement was presented and, through an "unrestricted grant," also paid for the publication of the *Primary Care Companion* supplement. Cephalon also has paid the lead authors of all eight papers in the supplement, either through honoraria, consultant activities, speaking engagements, or (in one case) research funds.[5] The *Primary Care Companion* is described as the official journal of the Association of Medicine and Psychiatry. This supplement is a shameful marketing tool.

Marketing by Doctors

It has been easy to recruit physicians to help pharmaceutical companies market their new drugs. Just send them to a resort, dub them consultants, and pay them. A case in point was the campaign by Searle (now Pfizer) to increase sales of their new pain reliever Celebrex. Searle recruited 300 physicians to come to Orlando for a weekend to learn about the drug. Searle paid their expenses and gave each $500 for attending. Those who were willing to give talks about Celebrex to other doctors for the company received $500 more for each talk. Around the same time Merck, in direct competition with Searle, paid physicians $1,000 as consultants to attend a one-day meeting in Boston about its new product.[6]

Another wrinkle in marketing, called to my attention by a faculty member at the University of California at San Francisco, was an invitation in 2001 to a talk at the house of a fellow faculty member about a new drug for hepatitis. The invitation contained no acknowledgment of the sponsor, but it displayed two logos: one of "Projects in Knowledge," an "Education Initiative in Gastroenterology," and Home Delivery CME, with its slogan, "Right Place, Right Time." The sponsor was, in fact, the Schering Corporation, which at the time (January 2001) was involved with drugs for treating hepatitis.[7] The faculty member who sent me the invitation remarked: "I was appalled to learn that a member of this faculty was willing to open her home to strangers in return for what must be financial and/or professional gain. In my opinion, this represents extraordinarily unseemly behavior."[8]

And here is another effort by academics that aids a company in marketing, but in this case it involves an academic office of CME. Early in 2003, one of my colleagues sent me a copy of a letter that invited him to speak for Berlex Laboratories. It turned out that Berlex had paid Health Learning Systems, a medical education company, to hire academic physicians to prepare a set of slides on heparin-induced thrombocytopenia, a specific complication of treatment with heparin (a blood thinner). Berlex has had a drug on the market for a few years (Reflutan) that effectively treats the complication. A competing drug for the same condition (Argatroban) is made by GlaxoSmithKline. Academic physicians at the University of Pennsylvania were paid several thousand dollars each to prepare a slide set about the condition. Health Learning Systems then offered $1,200 to each of 30 physicians to stay at the Ritz-Carlton Hotel in Phoenix, Arizona and learn how to use the slide set. Each physician would then be capable of using the slide set to give these talks at various hospitals and would be paid another $1,200 for each session.[9]

Seven of the eight academic physicians selected by the CME department at Penn to prepare the slide set had financial arrangements with Berlex, having earned money for consulting with the company or speaking for it.[10] They prepared the slides without interference by Health Learning Systems, though representatives sat in on the meeting when the slides were developed. The slide set, which considered the value of both drugs, Reflutan and Argatroban, was considered unbiased in an independent review at Penn. Nonetheless, I asked an expert on heparin-induced thrombocytopenia at another university to assess whether the slides were biased toward one drug or the other. He asked to remain anonymous, but his remarks were:

> Drug "R" [Reflutan] had been presented first, (if alphabetical, would have been second), had been promoted as the "first drug approved. . . .", a clinically non-significant fact, and had been presented as a dual site inhibitor, not a single site inhibitor, as was Drug "A" [Argatroban]. In other words, the clinical data was subservient to irrelevancies. So, my initial impression was that Drug R was being promoted slightly more than Drug A. Of greater concern was the implication that a drug was needed in every circumstance for every patient who ever is diagnosed even with potential HIT [heparin-induced thrombocytopenia], whether a clot was ever diagnosed. Also, the initial slides focused on Drug A (NO KNOWN ANTIDOTE) vs. Drug R (no available antidote, although means exist to improve. . . .). It would appear that there is a greater toxicity to A vs. R. My impression was that drug R was more promoted than A . . . On balance, I would say the audience would have however learned much about the subject, and would have used Drug R when challenged with the clinical problem, after hearing the talk.[11]

So, is the slide series biased in favor of Reflutan because it is a better drug than Argatroban or for reasons related to the financial conflicts of the physicians who prepared the materials? My expert may be correct that the audience probably learned much about the subject. Clearly, the information may allow physicians who hear these lectures to care for their patients more effectively, but through a chain, beginning with the academic physicians who prepared the material, to the university department that offers postgraduate credits for the physicians who participate in the lectures, the academics have become marketing agents for Berlex.

The expert who reviewed the materials for me went on to say: "I suppose the worst part of this is that even if none of the authors had a financial relationship, it is now impossible or hard to truly believe the data are balanced, even if they are. What a mess. . . ."[12]

I asked Dr. Zalman Agus, the head of CME at the University of Pennsylvania, why he chose faculty members who had a financial conflict of interest with the company that funded the educational program. He replied by e-mail, but when I asked him whether I could quote his answer, he replied, "Permission denied."[13] Should a medical school department of continuing education produce lecture materials for a drug company with faculty who may be encumbered by financial connections to the company? Is it worth the financial gain?

These several examples illustrate how industry engages physicians in their marketing efforts. In some instances the physicians are merely helping to sell products, but in others, the financial arrangements with industry may be inducing them to develop biased educational materials.

Ghostwriting

Medical journals publish many useful educational articles that summarize the latest facts about a disease or a treatment. The physicians who submit these articles gain prestige and often a small honorarium. Journals expect that authors of such articles adhere to a time-worn ethic, namely that they are the legitimate authors of the work. As it turns out, such is not always the case. As pharmaceutical companies rush to get their newest drugs into widespread use, some have promoted their products in papers ghostwritten by science writers for "thought leaders" and sent to journals for publication under the thought leader's name. In some instances these papers have also recommended off-label uses of drugs. Although the "author" sometimes changed the text somewhat, if the paper no longer satisfied the company's marketing purposes, the company simply didn't submit it for publication. Many such guest authors performed little or no review of the article. They just signed their names and sent it off to a journal. The process is well hidden, but some examples can be cited.

Dr. Jack M. Gorman at Mt. Sinai School of Medicine in New York published an analysis of the antidepression drug Lexapro in a journal called

CNS Spectrums. The article said that Lexapro, a Forest Laboratory drug, was superior to an existing Forest Laboratory drug Celexa. (A subsequent independent analysis reached a contrary conclusion.) Notably, Lexapro was chemically similar to Celexa, but Celexa would be losing its patent protection in two years. Forest Laboratories had depended on Celexa for a substantial fraction of its sales, but undoubtedly was hoping to convince practitioners to switch to Lexapro. The transaction is laden with conflicts of interest. Dr. Gorman was not only a paid consultant for Forest Laboratories, but he was the editor of the journal in which his report was published (and Forest paid to publish the paper).[14]

Another example. While the family of a man who shot and killed his wife, his daughter, and his granddaughter and then committed suicide two days after taking the anti-anxiety drug Paxil was locked in a lawsuit against SmithKlineBeecham, David Dunner, a neurologist at the University of Washington, Geoff Dunbar, an employee of SmithKlineBeecham, and Stuart Montgomery, a British neurologist, prepared a paper on the risk of Paxil. Their study, published in *European Neuropsychopharmacology* in 1995, indicated that there was no increased risk of suicide with Paxil compared to placebo, thus seeming to bolster the company's case. In later court hearings it turned out that Dr. Dunner, the senior author, had seen only summaries of the original data on which the conclusion was based, not the original data. When he was asked about his involvement in the study, he said, "My role in the paper was that the data were presented to us and we analyzed it [*sic*] and wrote it [*sic*] up and wrote references."[15] Whether his extensive relations with pharmaceutical companies that make psychoactive drugs had any influence on his willingness to play such a role in the publication of the Paxil paper is not known.[16]

More on the aggressive attempts to market Neurontin. As part of their campaign to market off-label uses of Neurontin, Warner-Lambert hired a for-profit medical education company that paid medical experts to be authors of ghostwritten articles about the beneficial effects of Neurontin for pain, migraine, and psychiatric disorders (at the time, it was approved only for certain kinds of seizures). Some doctors accepted $1,000 from the company to sign their names to medical articles on off-label uses of Neurontin for submission to neurology and psychiatry journals, even though the articles had been written by technical writers hired by the pharmaceutical company. According to documents filed in the litigation against Pfizer for illegal marketing of off-label uses of the drug, the medical education company sent a memo to Warner-Lambert that said, "[the company] has draft completed, we just need an author." They recruited Dr. John Pellock at Virginia Commonwealth University to be the paper's author.[17] Fortunately, the drug has few side effects, yet there is an "opportunity cost" of taking the drug: patients given Neurontin might have benefited from taking a drug that was known to be useful for their conditions.

How much ghostwriting is going on and how much the physicians who submit the ghostwritten manuscripts for publication participate in editing them is unknown: such efforts are well hidden. However, in 1994, Dr. Troyen Brennan at Brigham and Women's Hospital in Boston received a request to submit a ghostwritten editorial for a pharmaceutical company about the possible legal liability of physicians who prescribe antihistamine drugs that cause somnolence. He was sent copies of several ghostwritten editorials and articles, some of which had been published in peer-reviewed journals. The proposal would have required little work and paid well ($2,500). He refused the invitation and published his experience instead as a warning about the conflicts of interest in this practice.[18]

The comments of a ghostwriter are also revealing. Linda Logdberg, who decided to quit ghostwriting medical articles after more than 12 years, described the process as "marketing masquerading as science." She indicated that although some authors meticulously went over her drafts before signing their names to them, others made no changes and simply signed their names to the manuscripts. She also said that the companies that solicit medical authorities to sign their names to papers that they had not originated would readily drop one of these authorities if they were not sufficiently malleable. She called ghostwriting "advertising that calls itself education."[19]

Ghostwriting Plus

Recognizing that obesity was becoming a major health problem in the United States, Dr. Richard L. Atkinson, an obesity researcher and head of the Beers-Murphy Clinical Nutrition Center at the University of Wisconsin-Madison

Medical School founded the American Obesity Association (AOA) and became its president. The AOA was intended to be an advocacy organization for the millions of persons in this country with obesity.[20] Unfortunately, a major aspect of its advocacy appears to be for the diet-pill-producing pharmaceutical industry. In a 1994 *Chicago Sun Times* article, Dr. Atkinson was quoted as saying that it was time to stop thinking of obesity as a problem of willpower, and start thinking of it as a chronic disease that requires long-term treatment. At the annual meeting of the American Diabetes Association that year, he said, "Diet, exercise and behavior modification just don't work [in the] long term. They require people to do unnatural things. The time has come to start thinking about drugs, when current treatments of obesity have failed."[21]

AOA publicly admitted that it received most of its funding from major pharmaceutical companies that market diet pills including Roche Laboratories (makers of Xenical), Knoll Pharmaceutical (makers of Meridia), Wyeth Laboratories (makers of Redux and Pondimin), and Medeva Pharmaceuticals (makers of Phentermine). A widely distributed book of recommended treatments for obesity, published jointly by AOA and Shape Up America! was supported by American Home Products, the parent company of Wyeth-Ayerst. Atkinson's work has also been supported by Weight Watchers International.[22]

Before Xenical was approved by the FDA, both Dr. Atkinson and Mr. Downey, Executive Director of the American Obesity Association, testified on the effectiveness and safety of the drug.[23] In July 2002, AOA prepared a statement instructing people how to deduct the costs of weight loss and weight control programs from their taxes. The statement was published on Roche Laboratories' Xenical Web page![24] Dr. Atkinson has been a consultant and on speaker's bureaus of many of these diet-pill companies. He told one reporter that he had been a consultant for about 20 companies.[25]

Dr. Atkinson publishes extensively on obesity and its treatment. At the end of a 20-page article in the *Annual Review of Nutrition* in 1997 entitled, "Use of Drugs in the Treatment of Obesity" he indicated that the work had been supported by his Beers-Murphy Clinical Nutrition Center.[26] The Center does receive research support from the National Institutes of Health, but also has substantial funding from the diet-pill industry. In listing only the Beers-Murphy Center as support, the author essentially hid his industry funding.

Equally problematic was Dr. Atkinson's role as a ghostwriter in an article about drugs for obesity. Matthew Kauffman and Andrew Julien of the *Hartford Courant* newspaper discovered that Dr. Atkinson had been paid by the pharmaceutical company Wyeth-Ayerst to be the author of an article for a medical journal written by a science writer about the benefits and risks of Redux.[27] Atkinson claimed he didn't know that Wyeth-Ayerst had paid to have the article written. As it turned out, the article was never published; Redux was removed from the market because it was found to have life-threatening heart and lung complications. In response to the accusation that he had become a shill for drug companies, Dr. Atkinson said, "obviously I like to get paid. I like to have money. They have meetings sometimes in pretty nice places. I love that. That's great. But I really hope that I don't allow those relatively trivial and in many instances completely trivial material things to get in the way of science. That would be awful." Nonetheless, he mused, "I think I've been pretty honest and uncorrupted by the money. But who knows, maybe it's so insidious that I don't notice it."[28]

That he can be so blasé about this kind of activity suggests the degree to which doctors can lose their moral compasses. The Web site of the Center for Science in the Public Interest lists more than a dozen pharmaceutical, diet food, and weight loss companies for which Dr. Atkinson consults or lectures, as well as many more from which he has received research support.[29] Dr. Atkinson admitted that drug companies "love me" because of his strong support for the use of diet pills.[30] Was his judgment influenced by excessive closeness to industry with their perks and support? Perhaps only Dr. Atkinson knows.

"Chemo Is Our Cardiac Cath"

It's hard to imagine an illness that makes a person more vulnerable than metastatic cancer, the stage of the disease in which the tumor has become widespread throughout the body. People assume immediately that this diagnosis is tantamount to a death sentence (which it often is). Those who are afflicted reach out for even the most meager hope of escaping the ravages of the disease or prolonging their lives. They suffer not just from the disease but also from its aggressive treatment with chemotherapy. Life-threatening infections, sterility, uncontrollable diarrhea, harrowing nausea, hair loss, bleeding, and painful urination are well-known side effects of drugs that at once are trying to kill tumor cells but at the same time damage normal cells. The physicians best equipped and best able to treat such conditions are oncologists. Some are surgeons and surgical specialists such as gynecologists; most are subspecialists in internal medicine. The problem is that the structure of the reimbursement system for doctors who treat patients with metastatic cancer creates a financial conflict of interest that has a powerful influence on the physician and a potential for harm to these vulnerable patients.

In short, most practicing oncologists are paid on a fee-for-service basis. Until very recently, for an office visit alone, one in which the patient leaves only with a prescription for oral drugs, the doctor was paid approximately $60, a woefully inadequate payment for the necessary time to spend with a patient with a life-threatening illness and the overhead of running an office. If, instead, the doctor decided to give the patient an intravenous infusion of a chemotherapeutic drug (let us call it "chemo") to combat the tumor, an injection of a drug to prevent the severe nausea ordinarily brought on by the chemo, or an injection of another drug to boost the patient's flagging blood count, the doctor would have been paid several hundred dollars. Why the difference? Because oncologists, entirely within the law, purchase drugs for injection from distributors at the "average wholesale price" and sell it back to the patient or his insurer at a higher, retail price.[31] The idea of this arrangement is that the markup between wholesale and retail prices is expected to cover the oncologist's overhead associated with administering the drugs. The margin between wholesale and retail costs is quite different among drugs, making it more profitable for the physicians to administer some drugs than others. Moreover, the reimbursement is dose dependent. Until quite recently, reimbursement for an 8 mg dose of Zofran, a drug that substantially lessens the chemo-induced nausea and vomiting, yielded $25, and for 32 mg the reimbursement was $125. Some oncologists gave the larger dose even though the smaller dose is usually just as effective.[32] They pocketed the extra $100.

The possibility that the choice of drug was sometimes being made because of profits rather than optimal clinical judgment caught the attention of Congress. In a 2001 hearing on Medicare drug reimbursement in the House of Representatives, Representative James Greenwood made this comment: "We will hear how the profits available for utilizing certain drugs appear to be improperly affecting some health care providers' clinical decisions, influencing them to provide unnecessary care and utilize drugs based on profit margins rather than therapeutic efficiency. For example, we will learn of cases in which the utilization of certain drugs skyrocketed without any reasonable clinical justification after manufacturers created large Medicare-funded financial windfalls to health care providers to encourage them to use their drugs."[33]

How a patient with advanced cancer is treated depends on many factors, especially the type of tumor, its location, its histologic appearance, and extent of spread. Beyond these "medical" imperatives, however, are those related to the patient's own preferences for treatment and the doctor-patient interaction. Take three realistic scenarios in which a patient, newly diagnosed with metastatic lung cancer arrives in the office of an oncologist. In the first, the doctor explains the nature of the disease and estimates the patient's prognosis, describes the treatment options that are available (one of which is no chemo at all) including the expected side effects of treatment, and tries to engage the patient in making treatment decisions. Many oncologists recognize that even in their extreme anguish, most patients want to be informed and make their own choices. In this scenario, the patient and the family decide not to pursue further treatment, including chemotherapy.

But here is another realistic scenario: the patient, frightened about the disease and easily intimidated by a physician, is greeted by an oncologist who asserts that the patient has a limited life expectancy but studies show that certain drugs can prolong the lives somewhat of patients with like diseases. Perhaps the doctor underestimates the hazards of chemo or overestimates the patient's life expectancy, and believes that a course of chemo might help. One course of chemo is given, drugs to combat anemia are also administered, a short improvement occurs, and when the tumor recurs, another course of chemo is given. Meanwhile, the patient has suffered the ravages of chemotherapy, including severe nausea, vomiting, diarrhea, and hair loss, and the prolongation of his life, if any, has been difficult to endure. In a final scenario, a doctor is reluctant to administer chemo, knowing that the chance of a meaningful response is negligible, yet the family insists on "doing something."

In these scenarios, the doctor has great discretion over which course treatment takes. The second scenario (the most aggressive one), though it fails to involve the patient in decision making, is not wrong. It is not malpractice. In fact, a review of the course of treatment by another independent oncologist would probably show that the treating doctor's decision was appropriate. Nonetheless, there is a great temptation to bypass patient decision making, to go the chemo route, and to reap the financial rewards of aggressive therapy. The oncologist can easily convince himself that in treating aggressively, he is giving the patient the best chance; that the side effects of chemo are really not that bad, and that by treating the patient for anemia he is improving the patient's quality of life. Because the financial motive is there, but well hidden (possibly even to the doctor himself), treatment decisions like these are insidious. In fact, though ultimately the physician can often set the therapeutic agenda in individual patients, the reimbursement system itself makes these options possible. In addition, as the third scenario suggests, pressures from families to "do something" often play into the oncologists' decisions.

Nevertheless, the system is susceptible to abuse, and it has been abused. One oncologist half jokingly told me, "Chemo is our cardiac cath, or our arthroscopy," implying that chemo offers a profitable "procedure" for the oncologist analogous to the invasive procedures of other medical and surgical specialties.[34] Another oncologist criticized this arrangement as "the dirty little secret of oncology."[35] In 2002, the average income of oncologists was approximately $310,000, and some have a net income far greater.[36] Until this year, approximately two-thirds of the income of oncologists in community practice was derived from intravenous or intramuscular drugs.[37] Dr. Peter Eisenberg, an oncologist who practices in a ten-person group in Marin County in California, said that between two oncologists literally across the hall from each other, there may be substantial differences in the use of chemo for patients with advanced cancer. These differences, he averred, might be based only on differences in opinion about the best practice for their patients, on patients' expectations, on family demands, or even on the physician's deep desire to fight the disease to the end. Yet in some instances therapeutic decisions are made on the basis of reimbursement. Some oncologists, Dr. Eisenberg said, make an income of nearly a million dollars a year by pushing chemotherapy. He said, "the financial conflicts I have identified in our discipline . . . are so pervasive and insidious that we continually must remind ourselves as to the real purpose of our work."[38]

A study that received little attention when it was published in April 2003 raises additional questions about the rationale for chemotherapy. Based on a general concern that chemotherapy is being overused at the end of life, Ezekiel Emanuel, Norman Levinsky, and their colleagues examined the Medicare records of nearly 9,000 patients who died of cancer in Massachusetts and California. They discovered that "Chemotherapy use was similar for patients with breast, colon, and ovarian cancer [tumors that are known to be responsive to chemotherapy] and those with cancer generally considered unresponsive to chemotherapy, such as pancreatic, hepatocellular [liver], or renal-cell [kidney] cancer or melanoma." Why, they asked in their paper, are doctors treating patients when medical evidence indicates that there would be no benefit and only possible harm? They considered many possibilities, including demands for treatment by patients and families, providing time for patients to adjust to the shock of the bad diagnosis, and uncertainty about a patient's prognosis or a tumor's responsiveness.[39] They did not consider another possibility raised by the foregoing discussion, namely that physicians' financial incentives might have been a motivator in some cases.

It's important to note here that most oncologists work very hard, take care of the sickest patents, and have the awful experience of seeing a large fraction of their efforts fail and their patients suffer (sometimes horribly) and die. I do not begrudge them a good income, or even a large income, for the difficult, emotionally draining work they do. I do fault any, however, who take advantage of sick, worried patients and their anguished families by giving chemotherapy when they know the result will be futile, or manipulating the kind of therapy for personal financial reasons.

The possibility that oncologists are responsible for excessive costs has not escaped the attention of the federal government, which pays much of the bills in the Medicare program. In 2003, Medicare reduced payments for drugs but increased payments for office visits, keeping total reimbursement about the same. This change was met with anger by some oncologists, who argued that they might have to revert to using older, less effective drugs.[40] The risk, of course, is that cuts in reimbursement for these out-patient treatments will inhibit appropriate and necessary treatment and reduce the amount of time that oncologists need to spend with their patients to explain their prognosis and complex treatment regimens. If this happens, those who abused the system for personal gain will have caused great harm to many patients.

Not surprisingly, the pharmaceutical industry is quite content with the current arrangement, which if anything strongly favors the use of its products, and the industry mounted a lobbying campaign to preserve it. In fact, internal documents for one company show that some drug companies manipulated the market by lowering certain wholesale prices to physicians, which in turn increased the margin between the price that physicians pay and charge and thus encouraged oncologists to use more of their particular drug.[41] Such practices could now lead to serious penalties.

Selling Free Samples

Like oncologists, urologists also use injectable drugs that they buy at wholesale and sell to Medicare, other insurers, and their patients at a markup. Two roughly equivalent drugs for advanced prostate cancer, Lupron (TAP Pharmaceuticals) and Zoladex (AstraZeneca) are administered at intervals, at least monthly, in physicians' offices. Both drugs are an alternative to castration, which was the most effective treatment before these drugs were available. Urologists are free to prescribe either drug, and because (like chemotherapy drugs described before) they are administered by injection, Medicare pays the physicians directly for the drugs. Thus, depending on the difference between the price a company charged for the drug (the wholesale price) and the price that physicians charged insurers for administering it (the retail price), the drug with the largest margin between wholesale and retail prices could be chosen. Many urologists prescribed either Lupron or Zoladex, depending on which would provide the largest financial return. Unfortunately, in doing so, they often prescribed the more expensive drug,[42] thus costing Medicare and other insurers approximately

$30 million more than was appropriate.[43] By one estimate, one urologist with 30 patients under treatment with one of these drugs could earn about $50,000 per year from the drug alone. Some must have brought in much more: one physician billed more than $4 million for the drugs over a five-year period. "For example, in 1997, a year in which Medicare spent $504.1 million on Lupron, there were 14,316 urologists nationwide who submitted claims to Medicare for Lupron prescribed to patients. Of that number, 3.4 percent . . . received 25 percent of all monies paid out by Medicare for prescriptions for Lupron. . . . The top 25 of the urologists (3,574) received 82 percent, or $411.6 million, of the total $504.1 million."[44]

Urologists were also offered (and many accepted) substantial discounts on Lupron as an inducement to prescribe more of the drug. Throughout the 1990s, TAP gave out more than $7 million of value in free samples per year. Some urologists illegally billed the free samples to the insurers and to patients, and several ultimately pleaded guilty to Medicare fraud. Of course, many urologists, probably the majority, never billed for free samples. Many, however took part in other TAP inducements, described in the government's settlement summary as "off-invoice price discounts, all expense paid trips, 'educational grants,' payment of bar tabs, payment of holiday party expenses, financial support for advertising expenses, free consulting services, and forgiveness of debt [for previous drug purchases]."[45] It is noteworthy that the American Urological Association tried to get TAP to stop the practice of using free samples as a sales inducement, but TAP had no obligation to this professional organization and the practice continued on. In 2001, the illegal efforts by TAP Pharmaceuticals to induce physicians to use Lupron culminated in a payment by TAP to the federal government, all 50 states, and the District of Columbia of nearly 900 million dollars.[46]

TAP was not the only company that had to pay a fine for illegal sales practices. Its competitor, AstraZeneca, the manufacturers of Zoladex, subsequently paid the federal government $266 million for a similar practice.[47]

Selling Risky Dietary Supplements

Until quite recently, doctors across the country were purchasing dietary supplements that contain ephedra, a chemical stimulant, and were reselling it to

their patients as an aid to weight loss. Some of the same doctors were helping companies that make these supplements market them by allowing their
names to be used in company advertising. For these office sales they were
able to make as much as $250,000 per year. The problem is that ephedra-
containing supplements had been linked to many cases of cardiac arrest.
Although a causal link between the drug and this complication was not
definitive, over the past decade there were more than 100 deaths in people
using ephedra. Only recently the FDA removed the product from the market. Before this action was taken, however, some physicians tried to convince local authorities and even the Secretary of Health and Human
Services to keep ephedra-containing supplements on the market.[48] Notably, these are some of the same physicians who were profiting from selling
the supplements.

Helping Companies Avoid Lawsuits

In 1999 Dr. Baha Sabai, chief of the University of Tennessee's division of
maternal-fetal medicine, submitted a study for publication to the *American
Journal of Obstetrics and Gynecology* that purported to exonerate a drug called
Parlodel as the cause of strokes in women who had just given birth. Several
years earlier, Parlodel had been widely used to suppress lactation and thus
avoid the pain of swollen breasts after delivery for women who chose not to
breast-feed. Unfortunately Dr. Sabai's study was seriously flawed, and he
had substantial financial conflicts of interest with Sandoz Pharmaceuticals
(now Novartis), the company that makes Parlodel.

Dr. Sabai, (an obstetrician), had carved out neurologic consequences of
pregnancies, including eclampsia, as an area of expertise in the obstetrical
community. (Dr. Sabai has since moved to the University of Cincinnati.)
His study was about strokes in women after delivery. The defects in their
study probably would never have seen the light of day if Dr. Sabai and his
co-author, Dr. Andrea Witlin, had not been deposed by a keen lawyer for a
woman who developed a stroke after taking Parlodel. The paper reported
20 patients who suffered from serious strokes after they left the hospital
following childbirth. It said that there had been approximately 130,000 de-
liveries in the 20 years of the study, that 40,000 patients had taken Parlodel,

and that only one of these patients had suffered from a stroke. Sabai and Witlin concluded, among other things, that Parlodel was not a cause of strokes in the postpartum period.[49]

There was something odd about this conclusion when Drs. Sabai and Witlin submitted their manuscript for publication: Parlodel was no longer on the market for postpartum breast engorgement. The FDA had forced Sandoz to recall it for this use in 1994 after a handful of patients developed strokes while taking the drug. After their paper had been submitted for publication to the *American Journal of Obstetrics and Gynecology*, Drs. Sabai and Witlin received a favorable reply from the journal's editors and were about to resubmit their manuscript. At the time their conclusion about the possible relation between Parlodel and strokes was as follows: "Although bromocriptine [Parlodel] is no longer approved for use in postpartum lactation suppression . . . it does not appear to have been causal for postpartum stroke as has previously been reported. Instead it appears that its use may have been protective. Indeed, one might argue that women exposed to bromocriptine were at a lower risk for stroke than those women not receiving bromocriptine."[50]

The depositions of Drs. Sabai and Witlin, however, revealed several serious irregularities. First, Dr. Sabai had been a paid expert witness for Sandoz in suits involving Parlodel on several previous occasions since 1994 or 1995. He admitted that his payments had averaged $10,000 to $20,000 per year, and in one year was more than $20,000.[51] Despite the requirement of the *American Journal of Obstetrics and Gynecology* that authors reveal any commercial ties to companies whose products they are featuring in their manuscripts, Dr. Sabai did not do so.[52] Second, although the manuscript described the research as a prospective study, no data were kept on an ongoing basis as patients with strokes were seen. No written criteria were set at the beginning for including patients in the study. Missing data were sometimes patched in out of Dr. Sabai's memory.[53] The only data, which existed on a single floppy disk, could not be independently verified. The numbers 40,000 and 130,000 were simply estimates. In short, as the lawyer for the stroke patient argued, some of the data were incomplete, unreliable, unverifiable, and nonreproducible.[54]

Thus, five years after the drug was no longer available for breast engorgement, Drs. Sabai and Witlin submitted a seriously flawed study for publication that favored Sandoz' interpretation that Parlodel was not the cause of postpartum strokes. The final published version of the study omitted any discussion of Parlodel. Clearly the research of Drs. Sabai and Witlin was not only flawed, but contaminated by Dr. Sabai's financial conflict of interest.

Profiting From a Class-Action Lawsuit

In 2002, two expert cardiologists, Dr. Linda J. Crouse, of Kansas City and Dr. Richard Mueller of New York City, were severely criticized by the United States District Court in Pennsylvania for profiteering and inappropriate conduct in performing and reading echocardiograms and completing medical forms. The case involved 78 patients who were part of a class-action lawsuit against American Home Products (now Wyeth Laboratories) for damage caused by their products Pondimin and Redux. Defects in heart valves had been attributed to both of these drugs, and a properly performed echocardiogram is required to assess possible valve damage. After engaging several independent experts to review the echocardiograms that were considered by these two cardiologists to be indicative of moderate to severe damage (and thus rendered the patient eligible for remuneration in the lawsuit), the Court found: "that two cardiologists had made medically unreasonable judgments on a broad scale, that law firms retained cardiologists, and that one firm worked out a questionable financial arrangement with one cardiologist and was deeply involved with completing medical portions of forms for both cardiologists."[55]

The court made several assertions. Among them that both cardiologists had exaggerated the severity of the valve damage, misidentified normal flow across heart valves for valve malfunction, and both allowed one of two law firms to complete medical forms that they, by law, were required to complete. It said that Dr. Crouse allowed a law-firm employee to teach her echocardiography technician how to carry out the tests on the law-firm's patients so that the head technician "understood how to make the measurements." She received $1,000 for each of the 725 cases from one firm and $250 each for approximately 10,000 echocardiograms from another group of law firms, yielding an income of at least $2,725,000 for these tests alone in a period of less than a year. Notably, for the patients of the first firm, the court found that she allowed a representative of the law firm to be present in the office when their clients were being examined and that she never reviewed patients' medical records or examined any of the patients. The Court said that: "The circumstances under which the Dr. Crouse echocardiograms were performed and interpreted undermine her credibility. . . . Dr. Crouse spent little time actually reviewing and approving the results of these echocardiograms. . . . When considering the thousands of echocardiograms that Dr. Crouse interpreted during the period that she worked for the Hariton and Napoli firms, her practice resembled a mass production operation that would have been the envy of Henry Ford."[56]

The Court also criticized Dr. Mueller. Though he spent far more time with the clients of the Hariton firm than had Dr. Crouse, the Court found that he also allowed firm representatives to be in his office when the tests were done, he allowed law-firm representatives to complete medical forms that he later signed, he used testing procedures that exaggerated the degree of valve malfunction, and that his interpretations of the tests were "beyond the bounds of medical reason." Dr. Mueller was paid between $325,000 to $500,000 for his work. The Court was especially critical of a financial arrangement between the law firm and Dr. Mueller. It said: "Dr. Mueller stood to earn an additional amount when his echocardiogram reading showed moderate or severe mitral regurgitation [valve malfunction] . . . he received an extra $1,500 if the claimant obtained a benefit or the claim was submitted to the Trust [the settlement arrangement for the class-action suit] for payment. . . . Thus, Dr. Mueller's remuneration depended on how he interpreted the echocardiogram and on what he stated on the form. He had a financial incentive to reach a particular result."[57]

Finally, the Court concluded that most of the patients recommended by these two physicians for settlements from the Trust would have received large sums of money inappropriately, thus possibly depriving some patients who deserved compensation from receiving it. Both physicians have denied any impropriety, and the decision of the court has been appealed.

The extent of involvement of physicians in legal transactions, and the possible influence on them based on the party that pays their consulting fees is not known. It seems highly unlikely that the instances described here are isolated instances. It seems equally likely that financial ties do have an influence on judgments they offer.

Influencing NIH and FDA Decisions

Finding a treatment for diabetes is a worthy endeavor. Rezulin, a drug with effects on sugar metabolism different from the available drugs in the mid-1990s, seemed to be a promising addition to the medications then in use. Unfortunately, after only a little more than three years on the market, it had been linked to 63 deaths from liver failure; hundreds more treated with the drug developed liver dysfunction. By the time it was withdrawn from the market, however, Warner-Lambert (now a division of Pfizer) had sales of several billion dollars.[58] Financial conflict of interest was only one of the many factors that account for the misfortunes of the patients who were injured by the drug: pressure by Congress to speed up approval of new drugs, excessive kowtowing to industry by government officials, poor judgment by other officials in allowing conflicted scientists to participate in decision making, and aggressive attempts by the company to paper over the gravity of drug complications and to preserve sales all contributed. Nonetheless, financial arrangements between physicians and industry were important components. We owe the "inside information" to the dogged investigations of David Willman of the *Los Angeles Times*.

Rezulin was one of the drugs selected for the National Diabetes Prevention Study by the National Institutes of Health. Participants who were otherwise healthy received the drug in the hope that its action would prevent the development of the adult type of diabetes. From the very beginning of the study in June 1996, Warner-Lambert was involved: it had pledged to contribute about $20 million toward the expense of the $150 million study, which had hoped to enroll 4,000 subjects. Also from the beginning, important financial conflicts of interest had developed. Dr. Jerrold Olefsky, a highly regarded diabetes researcher, initially chaired the committee that selected Rezulin as one of the drugs to be tested. Dr. Olefsky, as it turned out, held three separate patents as the sole or first inventor of the drug, and was the founding co-chair of a Warner-Lambert–created and sponsored group called the National Diabetes Initiative. Subsequently, as a paid Warner-Lambert consultant, he spoke on behalf of Rezulin to the FDA Advisory Committee that approved Rezulin. Although Dr. Olefsky was later replaced as chair of the committee because of his evident conflicts, he was still allowed to remain on the study's steering committee.[59]

A second person with a substantial financial conflict of interest was Dr. Richard Eastman, who was then the NIH's top diabetes researcher with responsibility for the National Diabetes Prevention Study. Although government service generally precludes employees from having financial conflicts of interest, Dr. Eastman had ties not only with Warner-Lambert but several other companies as well, and his superiors had approved them. Dr. Eastman had accepted $78,455 from Warner-Lambert, was an advisor for Warner-Lambert, and was a speaker for a company-sponsored group that recommended that doctors use Rezulin for their patients.[60] Notably, a lawyer at the Department of Health and Human Services warned Dr. Eastman at the beginning of the study to recuse himself from all official matters involving Warner-Lambert or to divest all holdings if recusal substantially interfered with the performance of his duties. According to reporter Willman, Dr. Eastman continued to participate in discussions about Rezulin.[61]

As the study progressed, tests of liver function began to show nearly four times more liver injury in people who were taking Rezulin in the NIH study than those who were taking placebos. Warner-Lambert believed that the abnormalities would disappear once the drug was discontinued and that close monitoring by repeated testing would provide the signal to hold off giving it. This assumption later was found to be fatally incorrect.[62]

In parallel with the NIH study, the FDA was considering approving Rezulin for use by the nation's diabetics, and with the pressure from Congress to move new drugs through the approval process rapidly (and presumably to be more friendly to the pharmaceutical industry), the drug was approved after a shorter-than-usual review. Notably, it was approved over the strong objections of Dr. John Gueriguian, a veteran FDA medical officer, who had reviewed Rezulin's safety and effectiveness. Gueriguian was removed from the Rezulin review at Warner-Lambert's request before the FDA Advisory Committee's vote in December 1996 that, in turn, led to FDA approval in January 1997.

Shortly after Rezulin was approved for use by the nation's diabetics, it achieved wide use (by December 1998, sales were nearly $1 billion). Liver injury cases continued to mount, and in December 1997 the FDA's counterpart in Britain, the British Medicines Control Agency, removed the drug from the market there. When Audrey LaRue Jones, a healthy schoolteacher who had enrolled in the NIH study, died of liver failure in May 1998 despite close monitoring of her liver function, Rezulin was withdrawn from the NIH's National Diabetes Prevention Study. But it was not taken off the market immediately for diabetics. The FDA only required that Warner-Lambert warn doctors to test liver function more frequently. Between May 1998 when Ms. Jones died and March 1999, more deaths occurred from liver failure. In fact, up until December 1998, the FDA had reports of 33 deaths attributed to Rezulin.[63]

In January 1999, after the newly appointed FDA Commissioner Jane Henney took office, she called for reevaluation of Rezulin, and in March the Advisory Committee met again to consider what to do with the drug. The FDA, like other federal agencies, has well-defined conflict-of-interest regulations, but it can grant a waiver to "Special Government Employees" who have commercial ties that might influence them to serve on its committees under certain circumstances. In this case, nine of the ten physicians who reported on the safety and effectiveness of Rezulin at the March 26, 1999, meeting were paid Warner-Lambert consultants.[64] The committee voted 11 to 1 to keep the drug on the market.[65] Presumably, they must have thought that a small risk of serious complications was worth taking, given that the drug was effective for so many diabetics. Whether their connection to Warner-Lambert contributed to their opinion is not known.

One year later Rezulin was finally removed from the market. By then, 63 deaths from liver failure had been attributed to the drug. As of March 2003, nearly 9,000 suits had been filed by Rezulin users in various federal and state courts against Pfizer.[66]

The story is incomplete without mention of several heroes, including staff members at the FDA and physician researchers outside the FDA who tried to avert these tragedies. Among others, they include Dr. Gueriguian and Dr. Robert Misbin, who risked their jobs at the FDA to call attention to the risks of Rezulin.[67]

Shadowing

In 2002, a particularly egregious practice called "shadowing" came to light. In this practice, physicians were paid $350 to $500 per day by a pharmaceutical company to allow its representatives to stay in the doctors' offices as patients came and went.[68] In some instances the reps discussed the patient's treatment with the physician only after the patient was seen, but in others the drug representative was allowed to accompany the physician into the examining room. Some patients were not told who the visitor was. The doctors' collusion, while it may not be illegal, was certainly unethical. In 2003, a ruling by the Office of Inspector General makes it quite likely that shadowing is a practice of the past.

The examples described here show a profession heavily involved in helping industry market its products in speaking engagements, in ghostwritten articles, and in regulatory deliberations. They illustrate how some physicians exploit their professional standing to promote their own financial well-being over the best interests of their patients. Such actions harm patients, increase the cost of care, and deprive patients of appropriate compensation.

3

CONFLICTS OF INTEREST: FINANCIAL AND OTHERWISE

IN THE CONTEXT OF UNDERSTANDING HOW these complex financial relations with industry can lead to serious consequences for patient care, I have frequently referred to the notion of conflict of interest. Because conflicting interests are the basis for the kinds of adverse consequences described here, the nature and kinds of the conflicts must be defined clearly. In our context, a conflict of interest exists when a physician has dual and conflicting loyalties: on one hand to his professional responsibilities as a doctor, and on the other to his own personal welfare. Here we will be concerned primarily with conflicts that create a financial dilemma for the doctor, pitting the care of the patient against the financial well-being of the physician. Given that the physician has to make a living, it will be clear that such conflicts are inevitable and cannot be eliminated entirely, and as a consequence, the conflicts represent a condition in which a physician is in jeopardy of violating a trust.

Conflict of Interest: What Is It?

A conflict of interest exists when an individual or organization is in a position in which professional judgment concerning a primary interest tends to be unduly influenced by a secondary interest, such as financial gain.[1] It is a situation in which a personal interest conflicts with a demand of duty, in which regard for one duty tends to lead to disregard of another, or in which one duty tends to interfere with the proper exercise of judgment. Financial conflicts arise when an individual has competing interests that cannot be realized simultaneously, and where making a personal financial choice over a professional one could violate a code, a promise, or a professional responsibility. Conflicts of interest become a problem when there is a reasonable chance that a person will fail to fulfill an obligation to another.

Why the Fuss About Conflicts of Interest?

After all, I am not talking about overt corruption such as fraud, bribes, office-buying, or kickbacks. Yet what we are concerned about is equally problematic, far subtler, and largely hidden from sight. One observer commented: "Conflicts of interest are institutional weeds. They take root below the surface and become pervasive problems often long before they show their ugliness."[2] The weeds in this case expose physicians to powerful temptations to make money at the expense of their patients' welfare. Aside from harm to patients, conflicts of interest may be subconscious and as such can undermine judgment and integrity and lead to self-deception.

Conflicts of interest breed distrust. Because of financial conflicts of interest and even blatant hypocrisy in many nonmedical domains, the public is more suspicious and more cynical about those in public office, in business, in academia, in the clergy, and in the medical profession. Cynicism also abounds about the capacity of medicine to govern itself, and in several instances government agencies have had to promulgate rules or guidelines to correct inappropriate behaviors that the profession had not policed. For years, for example, we failed to enact sufficiently stringent ethical guidelines to stop kickbacks and self-referrals, and our history is scarred by failure to exclude from practice substandard practitioners and recalcitrant substance abusers. Our tendency in years past to use experience and judgment over medical evidence, our disregard of those few who wanted us to pay attention to the quality of care, and our failure to help restrain the cost of care were other factors that led many to question the medical profession's accountability, and in some instances, for state and the federal government to intervene.

Conflicts Promote Bias

Conflict of interest is often equated with bias, but in fact, it only unduly promotes bias; it provides no assurance that bias will result. Having a conflict of interest is not immoral or unethical. It is, however, unethical to act on the conflict in a way that cannot be justified ethically and thus violates a trust. Nonetheless, just because a physician stands to gain financially from some recommendation is not evidence that his motivation was necessarily pecuniary. A gastroenterologist, for example, may prefer colonoscopy over less expensive testing of the stool for blood, a cardiologist may do more many office tests than others, a urologist may recommend surgery for prostatic cancer over other treatments, and a lung specialist who carries out clinical trials on a drug may tout the benefits of the drug lavishly. In each case, the doctor has a financial incentive and thus has a conflict of interest. But, what motivates the doctor? The gastroenterologist has probably seen patients in the late stage of colon cancer when they cannot be saved, and he legitimately wants to protect people from getting cancer. He may never have considered that he might get more money from performing colonoscopy. The cardiologist may not have the same confidence in the clinical diagnosis of coronary disease as his peers, and pursues more testing than others because he wants to be more confident in the diagnosis of coronary disease before subjecting the patients to further invasive testing or to treatments. His only goal may have been proper diagnosis and treatment, not the added income from performing the tests. Given the state of knowledge about the treatment of prostate cancer, the urologist may believe that the results of surgery are better than seed implantation (and vise versa for the radiation oncologist). Neither might have considered whether he gets paid as a criterion.

How do we know whether their motives were based on their desire for income or the explanations listed here? The answer, of course, is that even when the action and the financial incentives are perfectly aligned, as they are in these examples, we do not know. We simply cannot crawl into the doctor's consciousness and extract the "true" explanation or motivation for their actions.

Detecting Bias

Unfortunately, it is not easy to detect bias in lectures or written material, and unless the physician is an expert in the field, it may be nearly impossible to do so. Subtle biases are particularly difficult to detect. A personal experience I had when I was editor of one of the most reliable medical journals, the *New England Journal of Medicine*, illustrates this point. In the mid-1990s former surgeon general C. Everett Koop announced that an epidemic of obesity was sweeping the nation.[3] At around that time a combination of two drugs, phen-fen (phentermine and fenfluramine) was being used widely off-label for weight loss. In the mid-1990s the FDA approved Redux (dexfenfluramine), a drug similar to fenfluramine, for weight loss and it also started to reach wide use.

In 1996, in the August 29 issue of the *New England Journal of Medicine*, we published an account of a serious complication of treatment with Redux: a small number of people who took the drug had developed a fatal or near-fatal disease of the lung's blood vessels (pulmonary hypertension).[4] Because of the diet drug craze at the time, we invited two well-known researchers, Dr. JoAnn Manson from Harvard Medical School and Dr. Gerald Faich at the University of Pennsylvania to write an accompanying editorial to put the complication in perspective. They wrote that drug treatment of obesity has its dangers, but they also cited the dangers of obesity, and they finally concluded that the risk of taking diet pills was less than the risk of remaining obese.[5]

Within hours after the commentary was published, the press reported that both Drs. Manson and Faich had been paid consultants for companies that stood to gain by selling diet pills, and a loud outcry ensued: the *New England Journal of Medicine* had violated its own rules and allowed someone with ties to the drug industry to write a commentary about the company's drug! Editorials condemning the *Journal*'s editors and the authors of the editorial appeared within days in the *Boston Globe*, the *Boston Herald*, the *New York Times*, and the *Atlanta Constitution*. The headline in the *Boston Globe* editorial on September 1 read, "Malpractice at a Medical Journal?"[6]

Among other things, it said: "A recent flap at the *New England Journal of Medicine* shows that even the most esteemed doctors can mix equal parts ethical and managerial lapses to damage the image of integrity essential to their profession. . . . Between the bungling and the dodging, no one emerges unsullied." It was true that we had violated our own rules, but it was unintentional: as it turned out, Dr. Manson's ties to the company were minimal, but Dr. Faich had been an ongoing consultant. But what about the Manson-Faich commentary? Was it biased?

It cautiously recommended treating obesity with drugs despite the risks. The conclusion read: "Obesity is an escalating problem in the United States, and the condition is notoriously difficult to treat. Because the associated health hazards are considerable, medications are needed that produce and maintain weight loss safely and effectively. Dexfenfluramine [Redux] is an important new drug in the clinician's arsenal, but it is not free of risk. Although physicians and patients need to be informed, the possible risk of pulmonary hypertension associated with dexfenfluramine is small and appears to be outweighed by benefits when the drug is used appropriately."[7]

When I first read the commentary, I was impressed with its careful evaluation of the costs and benefits of the treatment: risks of obesity on the one hand and benefits and risks of long-term diet drugs on the other. But after I knew that both authors had a financial conflict of interest, I read the commentary once more. On this second time through, I was not sure it was evenhanded. Neither was I sure that it was intentionally biased toward drugs, though this had nothing to do with the way it was written. Given the authors' reputations, it probably was their honest opinion about the trade-off between obesity and diet pills. The problem was that now that I knew about their relation to the drug industry, I had the seed of a doubt. Because of this experience, we tightened our rules so that we could try to avoid having anyone with a financial stake in a company (or a competing company) to write such commentaries.

Why Focus Only on Financial Conflicts of Interest?

Conflicting interests come in all sizes and shapes, and they are based on numerous subjective feelings, affiliations and associations, loyalties, prejudices, and experiences. Each creates a potential ideological or psychological impairment to an individual's judgment. Other factors that create conflict are moral beliefs, and a desire for power, prestige, or career advancement. Even zeal to create controversy, and animus against certain persons can be a motivator. Intellectual concepts can also induce powerful conflicts of interest: scientists develop a hypothesis based on their work and these hypotheses motivate them to push their ideas forward with further experimentation.

Sometimes, however, they tenaciously adhere to these hypotheses even when their experiments and those of others begin to prove that the concepts are inadequate or incorrect. In such instances advocacy, obsession, and passion can overwhelm sound judgment. The annals of science are filled with examples in which stubborn adherence to one hypothesis impeded another that later proved to be correct.

Note that all of these potentially motivating items are exclusively subjective, and although we might guess the intentions of a given person at any given time, we cannot be sure unless he acts in an overt fashion that exposes his bias. As noted before, not even the individual may know for sure what motivates him. These subjective conflicts can have powerful effects on people, but whether they have more or less influence than money undoubtedly varies. What is certain is that people have great difficulty ridding themselves of subjective conflicts and for that reason, one of the solutions to financial conflicts of interest, namely divestiture, cannot work for emotional or intellectual prejudgments. As Andrew Stark points out: "Compared with disclosing a pecuniary [financial] interest . . . disclosing a psychological bias comes far closer to admitting an irremediable incapacity to make an unencumbered decision."[8]

All of these conflicts of interest are intrinsic to an individual's beliefs, and they are not easily changed. Financial conflicts, however, have powerful influences, and they are optional: an individual can choose to have a financial conflict or to avoid one. Importantly, financial conflicts are identifiable, measurable, and susceptible to public disclosure and regulation. The promise of even modest financial gain can have a profound influence. Thus, it may be most prudent to assume that even for minor amounts, money (or a gift) represents a substantial motivator, and that a gift and the "return favor" can be disproportionate. Given this assumption, even pens, coffee cups, and a slice of pizza qualify as possible instigators of return favors. It is fair to point out that not everybody agrees. One scholar of conflict of interest makes the point that it is possible to carry financial conflicts of interest to the extreme. He said, "would we really expect a physician to jeopardize her job and her family's security for the most marginal of benefits to a patient, or to prevent the most trivial of harms?"[9]

Needless to say, it is not possible to prevent people from having encumbered states of mind based on the subjective perceptions described before, but because money is identifiable and fungible, circumstances where money is involved can be avoided or banned.

What About the Appearance of Conflict of Interest?

Many reports on conflict of interest lump together overt conflicts of interest and the appearance of conflict of interest, as if they are the same. By definition, someone who appears to have a conflict of interest does not necessarily have one, and yet is perceived as having one. As is the case for beauty, appearances of conflict of interest are strictly in the eye of the beholder. One observer describes this difference as follows, "Apparent conflicts of interest are no more conflicts of interest than stage money is money."[10] Nonetheless, the consequences to an individual who is suspected of having a conflict of interest, especially a financial one, can be serious, as the following example of Dr. Grossman illustrates. Someone can be eyed with suspicion when, in fact, they may be guilty of nothing. Considering apparent conflicts as true conflicts holds a person "hostage to the most cynical and suspicious elements of public opinion."[11]

Even though there is nothing improper or immoral about the appearance of conflict of interest, a widespread belief that someone has a financial conflict can have personal and political ramifications. The perception of wrongdoing can damage a person's reputation even though the individual may be completely innocent. I encountered a specific incident in the course of research for this book that illustrates this point. A cardiology colleague sent me a four-page, glossy, fold-out pamphlet from Vasomedical Inc., a company that makes a machine designed to treat angina. Though I was not familiar with the company, I was familiar with Dr. William Grossman, the chief of the Cardiology Division at the University of California at San Francisco, whose smiling face adorned two pages. On the front page, Dr. Grossman was quoted to the effect that he believed in the clinical usefulness of the machine made by the company. This quote and the subsequent interview with Dr. Grossman in the pamphlet seemed the epitome of a paid promotional statement, and my suspicions of financial conflict of interest were aroused. I sent Dr. Grossman an e-mail message gently asking him why a person of his stature and reputation would allow the company to "use" him that way. I also asked him whether he had a personal financial relation with Vasomedical. His reply follows:

You raise some important issues . . . First, I have absolutely no personal financial relationship with Vasomedical; no stock, no honoraria, no speaker fees, no air tickets, no hotel bills or meals, nothing! . . . I am very excited about EECP (the method pioneered by the company) as a non-invasive way of achieving marked improvement in coronary artery perfusion and ventricular unloading. . . . I had thought that some/most of the improvement that I have seen in my patients [treated with EECP] might well be placebo effect until I saw the data that Dr. [Andrew] Michaels obtained in the Cath Lab . . . the physiologic basis for improvement is much more plausible to me at this point. . . . When Vasomedical asked me if they could interview and photograph me for a promotional piece about EECP I hesitated (for fear of reactions like yours) but I decided to go ahead because I think this is a new and valuable treatment for our patients . . . and I would hate to see this small start-up company go under before the full therapeutic potential of their device is tested.[12]

In summary, Dr. Grossman's rationale had to do with his desire to improve patient care, not from any financial ties to Vasomedical. My initial perception of Dr. Grossman's motives was changed by his reply, yet others who are not aware of his motivation may well have had the same initial reaction as mine. Dr. Grossman's reply indicates that he knew that such interpretations were possible, and he was willing to take that risk. If the brochure had stated that Dr. Grossman had no financial ties to the company, it would have been clear that he was only performing a service by calling attention to a new, potentially useful treatment.

When extrapolated to the profession as a whole, it is quite apparent that perceptions of conflicts of interest can jeopardize public trust if large numbers of physicians are thought to be on the take. For this reason, avoiding even the appearance of conflict of interest tends to preserve public confidence in the judgment of a group or a profession.

Institutional Conflicts of Interest

The death of 17-year-old Jesse Gelsinger in 1999 during a gene-therapy experiment at the University of Pennsylvania brought the notion of institutional financial conflict of interest into sharp public focus. The teenager had a rare genetic disorder of metabolism, but he had done well on a special diet and medications. Mr. Gelsinger volunteered for the experiment even though he knew that he would not benefit personally from it. Unfortunately, the boy reacted badly to the virus that carried the new genes into his body and died unexpectedly. In the course of litigation over the death, a serious financial conflict of interest was uncovered. In essence, a financial benefit might have accrued not only to the clinical investigators, but also to their institution if their studies improved the fiscal welfare of a company in which the principal investigator and the institution had an equity share. It was subsequently revealed that inventors at academic medical centers and other institutions were also developing products and testing them in their own institutions, sometimes on their own patients. In the aftermath of this tragedy, the federal government temporarily shut down clinical research activities at many major medical centers.

During negotiations for a multimillion-dollar grant with a drug company for a clinical trial of the company's drug, a clinical researcher in Boston who wishes to remain anonymous insisted on maintaining control of the primary data, but the pharmaceutical company with whom he was collaborating continued to "play hardball" with its unwillingness to supply a copy of the original data to the researcher. Instead, the company only provided summaries of the data, which they had accumulated in the company's computers. At the same time, officers of the investigator's institution, eager to capture the substantial overhead from the grant, were pressing the researcher to relent on his requirement for data control. To bolster his case for preserving control of the data, the investigator contacted the two major journals that might eventually publish his study and received their assurance that they would consider publishing his study only if the researcher had access to all the data. The assurances he received helped him in his negotiations with the company.

Why are institutional arrangements such as these problematic? Simply put, they put leaders of academic medical centers and medical schools in a conflicted situation. These individuals have a vested interest in the success of their staff and faculty in converting their scientific discoveries into profitable inventions and products. Some institutions are already making millions of dollars in licensing the patents from this research, and many others are scrambling to cash in on these royalties at the same time that income from their faculty practices and other sources dwindles. Though their financial conflict of interest is not personal (the leaders do not generally pad their own wallets with such arrangements), patenting their faculty's inventions can be a substantial source of cash for the institution. Moreover, the research often produces tests and treatments that benefit patient care. Inhibiting faculty research based on concerns over financial conflicts of interest, therefore, can be counterproductive. The willingness of research professors, clinical investigators, and medical-device developers to develop potentially marketable inventions is likely to be curtailed if the inventors cannot expect to profit personally. Despite the purest of motives, academic leaders may be tempted to free up their faculty members to patent inventions and help market the resulting products. From the academic standpoint, this distribution of their faculty members' time and energy may not be in the best interests of the institution's academic mission. If they rein in the faculty because of worry about financial conflicts, we may be asking them to act in ways that are counter to the financial well-being of the institutions that they head. This is in itself, a difficult conflict for them.

A Flagrant Institutional Conflict of Interest

A specific example might help illustrate how an institution can have a profound financial conflict of interest. Shortly after Dr. Nancy Olivieri published favorable results of a treatment to remove excess iron from the body of heavily transfused children with thalassemia (a hereditary cause of anemia), she began to have concerns that the treated children were developing a complication from the drug involving the liver. When her concern reached high levels, she told officials at Apotex, the pharmaceutical company that sponsored the study, that she wanted to report her findings to her local institutional review board at the Hospital for Sick Children in Toronto. Apotex disagreed with her interpretation of the information and turned down her request. It cited a contract she had signed with the company and warned that, "information, whether written or not, obtained or generated by the Investigators during the period of the . . . contract and for a period of one year thereafter, shall be and remain secret and confidential and shall not be disclosed in any manner to any third party except with the prior written consent of Apotex . . . Apotex will . . . pursue all legal remedies in the event that there is a breach in these obligations."[13]

Olivieri, concerned about the patients' welfare, informed the review board anyway and published the results showing that the drug might be harmful. Apotex terminated the study at the Hospital for Sick Children and removed her from the study's steering committee, saying that they, "could not justify Nancy as the principal investigator in studies of a drug that she does not believe works."[14]

The responses of the Hospital for Sick Children and the University of Toronto were noteworthy. Instead of coming to Dr. Olivieri's defense, both institutions disavowed legal involvement (Dr. Olivieri had made the mistake of signing the contract without approval from either institution), refused to support her against any suits by Apotex, and removed her as the director of the program for treatment of the blood disease at the hospital.

In addition, a review committee appointed by the hospital blamed Dr. Olivieri for the mess[15] (though a committee appointed by the Canadian Association of University Teachers exonerated her).

Only later it was learned that the Hospital for Sick Children had been negotiating with Apotex, the largest pharmaceutical manufacturer in Canada (and the largest charitable donor in Canada) for a ten-million-dollar gift. Moreover, at the same time, the University of Toronto was negotiating with Apotex for a twenty-million-dollar grant to build a biomedical research center.[16]

Apotex erred by trying to keep possible drug toxicity confidential. Dr. Olivieri erred by not having the contract reviewed by the hospital or university and by signing the contract. And what about the hospital and university? Were the decisions not to support her, to blame her, and to remove her from her administrative position motivated by institutional conflict of interest? Many thought so.

Professional Organizations on the Take

More and more, medical professional organizations have become dependent on industry, especially the pharmaceutical industry, for financial support. They solicit support to subsidize their meetings, to fund grants and awards, and also use the funds to support their operations. Given the clout that such organizations have with their members, the pharmaceutical companies are eager to give the organizations large sums of money. When the company grants are unrestricted and completely untied to any society activity, there is little impact, but unencumbered gifts are rare. The issue is what professional societies "pay" for the largesse of industry. Some societies allow the companies to decide which lectures in a meeting they can sponsor, and which written or stored material (for example, lectures on CD-ROM) will carry a company's logo. Some societies give out the full demographic information on their members in exchange for a payment. The relations between the companies and the leaders of medical professional organizations are well hidden, but there is little doubt that the leaders of these professional organizations are acutely aware of which companies contribute financial support to ongoing programs. Professional organizations argue that their members would not be able to afford their dues or to attend their meetings without these subsidies, and that the subsidies do no harm. Such assurances are difficult to accept.

Shades of Gray

Are all conflicts of interest characterized by the same degree of potential unscrupulousness or do some practices produce more venal outcomes than others? Just as the law recognizes degrees of crimes, so too are the consequences of individual physicians' conflicts of interest. At my request, Neil Smelser, a prominent sociologist, laid out his views of a progression, from (as he described it) "not-so-bad" to "very bad." Generally, I agree with his rankings:

1. Being extra careful to cover oneself out of fear of loss through malpractice actions. This is often surely wasteful, but in many cases it would coincide with the wishes of the patient, and might cut down on taking shortcuts and careless practices. Everyone, including physicians, must be expected to protect oneself.
2. Working the system by undertreating (taking shortcuts to maximize the number of patients seen) or overtreating (too many unnecessary

tests, too many visits). This is worse than No. 1 because one is putting one's interest ahead of the patient, though the results may not necessarily be bad treatment.

3. Taking gifts from interested parties, because they create the presumption that the physician will favor the interests of those companies and his own interest at the same time, which of course does not put the patient first.

4. Actually undertaking behavior (e.g., using or pushing a certain medication) on behalf of agents who are entertaining, giving money to, or giving gifts to the physician. This is the next [worst] step, because one is actually acting in accord with the outside influence (rather than giving off the presumption that he/she might).

5. Engaging in bad practice (including harming patients) by following the dictates of one's own financial interest or those of persons in whose debt the physician is.[17]

Conflicts occur when competing interests cannot be realized simultaneously, and in this context, where making a personal financial choice over a professional one would violate a trust. Financial conflicts are troublesome because it is often extremely difficult to determine whether a conflicted person has been affected by the arrangement. Financial conflicts involve not only individuals but also institutions and professional organizations. The size of the financial inducement has some bearing on how nettlesome the conflict can be.

4

INFLUENCED BY GIFTS? NOT I!

Pʜʏsɪᴄɪᴀɴs' ꜰᴇʀᴠᴇɴᴛ ʙᴇʟɪᴇꜰ ᴛʜᴀᴛ ɪɴᴅᴜsᴛʀʏ-supported dinners, gifts, and trips do not influence them is based, in part, on their training designed to imbue a strong sense of objectivity. Students in medical school and house officers in postgraduate training are indoctrinated in the scientific method, which emphasizes a dispassionate approach to information. And in the last decade they also have been imbued with an almost religious adherence to "evidence-based medicine," a rigorously objective ascertainment of medical facts that involves standardized data collection and analysis. Thus, many physicians believe that they have no difficulty separating the facts from the hyped information given to them by industry representatives.

"It's educational," some doctors who participate in drug-company-sponsored lunches have told me. "I have to eat lunch anyway." "How else in my busy schedule would I get up-to-date information about the latest drugs?" "Why not take advantage of the companies' largesse—the industry is one of the most successful in the world and they have deep pockets." "I can't be bought, and even if there is a potential that I could be influenced in the drugs I prescribe, I take gifts from so many that I can't even remember which one gives me what." In one survey study, fewer than half of a group of 248 full-time faculty who were asked about the influence of free drug samples, subsidized education, and various meals and gifts believed that these gifts influenced their prescribing practices.[1]

What should we make of these often sincerely stated professions of objectivity? Before trying to understand the basis for their belief that they are invulnerable to influence, it may be worthwhile to examine a few specific reactions.

A Sample of Reactions

When I was editor of the *New England Journal of Medicine*, I published an opinion piece by Dr. Douglas Waud, a University of Massachusetts professor of pharmacology entitled, "Pharmaceutical promotions . . . a free lunch?"[2] Waud asked: "So where does one draw the line? I suggest that we simply not be on the take, whatever the amount or context. . . . I do not like the idea of a monetary limit on bribes (unless it is zero). Nor do I see the subsidization of education as appropriate. I believe that physicians can buy books and attend meetings without fear of landing in the poorhouse. I also don't buy the argument that asks, Would you be willing to have these arrangements generally known? My motivation comes from within, not from a fear that the *Boston Globe* may be looking over my shoulder."

A huge response to his criticism followed. Some of the responses were along the lines of the following:

> Do not . . . insult my intelligence or my integrity by claiming that I can be bribed into inappropriate professional behavior because of a free lunch.[3]

Another remarked:

> The government is encouraging the private sector to take a greater role in [continuing education] to save tax money. What little equity internists of my generation may have had is also eaten up by falling real estate values and increasing taxes. If the pharmaceutical companies do not help us, who will?[4]

Still another responded:

> The idea that accepting a shirt pocket protector valued at 50 cents will sway the judgment of a division chief is patently absurd. I find Dr. Waud's reference to what is appropriate behavior in this regard totally judgmental and narrow minded. His reference to the Hippocratic oath is most ill conceived. Several of its passages are no longer appropriate for conscientious physicians in the late twentieth century. Furthermore, the oath makes no reference to guarding the patient's financial well-being.[5]

These responses illustrate many different attitudes: a belief by physicians that they cannot be swayed, a view that company largesse is an adequate substitute for income from patient care and hostility to applying an ethical construct to matters of gift acceptance.

A decade later a director of medical education in a community hospital received a scathing letter from one of his "best internists," who was offended by a lecture I gave at his hospital about financial conflict of interest. He paraphrased the internist's complaints as follows:

[The internist] noted that your . . . presentation . . . created an emotional response among the physicians greater than any he has seen in the past two decades. This doctor was insulted by the implication that physicians can be corrupted with trivial gifts or free meals. In fact, since the intent of the drug-sponsored dinner lecture is clear at the outset (i.e. pharmaceutical marketing), sitting through an obvious marketing lecture was considered by this physician as appropriate "payment" in kind for the meal. I thought that the most interesting of his remarks focused on the context of pharmaceutical marketing to physicians in the greater world of business practice in this country. This physician asks why we, as physicians, agonize so much about the ethics of what are standard business practices in other industries. Sky boxes at sports arenas, high-priced restaurants, and luxury hotels all survive as means for providing business to business perks. Even the IRS recognizes the validity of "business entertainment" as a standard part of doing business by allowing travel and entertainment as tax deductions. This physician asks whether fast-food advertising in elementary schools (to an unsophisticated audience) is any more ethical than giving medical students medical instruments. Since we, as physicians, are not being treated by payers as professionals but only as line "providers" of health care services, why should we hold ourselves to values different than any other businesses?

My correspondent continued:

[This physician] questions why we, as physicians, should continue to provide services 24/7 and debate 80-hour work weeks when others only take advantage of our largesse and professionalism. In this context of feeling personally exploited, the few perks and sense of being valued remaining to a practicing physician are available from the pharmaceutical industry.[6]

The last comment is profoundly disappointing. People go into medicine with their eyes open, knowing that they will work hard and that part of the "return on their investment" of long years of study and low wages is not monetary, but satisfaction of helping people through difficult times. The comment also ignores the powerful influences of company-sponsored medical education. As Marianne Mattera, the editor of the magazine *Medical Economics* reminds us, "your prescriptions can be bought."[7]

Finally, here are a few more comments. After the disclosure that C. Everett Koop, former surgeon general, had supported extending the patent protection for Claritin (one of the first nonsedating antihistamines), but had accepted a million-dollar grant for the Koop Foundation from Schering-Plough, then Claritin's manufacturer, Dr. Koop said: "I have never been bought. I cannot be bought. I am an icon, and I have a reputation for honesty and integrity, and let the chips fall where they may. . . . It is true there are people in my situation who could not receive a million-dollar grant and stay objective. But I do."[8]

In a letter to the editor of the *Boston Globe* in 2002, neurologist Paul Rizzoli said:

> To me as a medical specialist, medications are tools. New medications are new tools; who better to hear from than the maker? I do not necessarily believe every claim by the new-car salesman, and I am certainly not brainwashed by the new-drug salesman. If the salesman values my time with some [gift] consideration, I don't see a problem. . . . Does the public really think that physicians are so stupid as to be bought by a dinner, prescribe based on our stomachs or wallets, or controlled by a sales pitch? Does it make sense that we would put into jeopardy our licenses, years of postgraduate education, residency, and specialty training, and years of patient care and established relationships, all for a dinner or a consultant fee?[9]

Medical Economics also reported that a physician quit the American Medical Association (AMA) over the issue of accepting gifts. As it turns out, the

AMA's restrictions on gifts are not severe, yet the physician said: "It's an insult to think that I would prescribe a drug just because I went on a trip or dinner to learn about it. . . . If a drug is good, helps my patients, and is economical, I will use it. Otherwise, I won't."[10]

And after the *ACP Observer*, an American College of Physicians newsletter, published a piece critical of the sales pitches of pharmaceutical representatives, Dr. C. R. Barksdale of Montgomery, Alabama, wrote: "I find it hard to believe that the profession, the government, or anyone else thinks it is wrong for drug companies to try to influence the sales of their products by 'feathering' the nest of physicians. Isn't that the American way? Every time I turn on a golf tournament, all the golfers wear advertisements. Baseball players, football players, movie stars, retired presidents—they all get paid to push some product. All those dollars spent run up the cost to consumers. How is that different from drug companies buying expensive meals? I hope *ACP Observer* will stay away from this topic and try to instead find some help in getting us paid at a fair rate."[11]

Examining These Responses

This sample of comments exposes an interesting range of hostile reactions. Some physicians genuinely believe that they cannot be influenced, and some of them are defensive or downright arrogant in their responses. Some have told me that drug companies are just there to help them and that they believe that the information they provide is accurate and unbiased. Some say that they are completely aware when drug company salesmen are trying to influence them and that they can resist the influence. One physician said that the drug reps can buy access but not loyalty (this is a frequent line from the drug companies). At one end of the spectrum are individuals who have a substantial monetary tie to a company, but whose conscious defenses are such that they try assiduously not to allow the money to influence their judgment. Such people might even "bend over backwards" in decision making to allow for complete fairness involving the products of the company with which he has ties.

A few of these responses highlight physicians' frustration about their financial and professional status. Both of these factors probably contribute to a greater willingness of physicians to become engaged in financial ventures with industry. Others admit that they take advantage of industry's deep pockets. Chances are that some have never even thought much about it: taking gifts, getting paid for speaking for a drug company, or going to a resort as a consultant has become the norm among their colleagues, and they assume that there's nothing wrong with it.

In Fact, They Can Be Influenced

Thus far I have referred to the trinkets and meals that pharmaceutical representatives hand out to physicians as "gifts." Because the gifts are motivated by the giver's motivation to sell a product, they are in reality marketing ploys, intended at a minimum to ingratiate the drug representative to the doctor, perhaps to raise awareness of certain products, and at the other extreme to create a sense of indebtedness. Such indebtedness is problematic because the physician's obligation to the drug salesman or his company often conflicts with his obligation to his patients.

Contrary to the introspective opinions of most physicians, but consistent with common sense, studies show that physicians *are* influenced by gifts and pharmaceutical promotions. The prescribing practices of physicians have been examined in a few studies in relation to some kind of exposure to a drug-company promotion. In one, 40 physicians who requested additions to their hospital's drug formularies (drugs carried and approved by their hospital) were compared to 80 who had not requested any new drugs. Statistically, doctors who requested the additions were 9 to 21 times more likely than those who did not to have eaten free meals from the companies, to have accepted drug-company money to attend or speak at a company-sponsored symposium, and to have accepted research support from the drug companies.[12] An independent review (in the same study) indicated that the newly requested drugs had little or no advantage over drugs already available. Another study of the prescribing practices of ten physicians who had attended company-supported symposia in resort locations showed a two- to threefold increase in the physicians' use of the drugs in the months after their trips.[13] Interestingly, a majority of physicians attending the symposia claimed that they would not be influenced by the enticements. Other studies confirmed the strong influence of drug representative interactions and gifts on the requesting of additions to hospital drug formularies.[14] The drug companies certainly are convinced of the existence of these powerful influences.

The acceptance of gifts and the obligations they create has complex motivations. Some insights can be drawn from common views of human nature and others from studies in psychology.

The Obligation of Reciprocation

Psychologists believe that reciprocation is one of the most powerful instruments of influence in our society. The "rule of reciprocation" states that we should try to repay, in kind, what another person has provided to us. Such a gift obligates us to a future repayment of items such as favors, gifts, and invitations. Psychology professor Robert Cialdini infiltrated groups of salespeople, fund-raisers, advertisers, and public relations firms to observe how such individuals use their persuasive tactics. He found that reciprocation for favors, development of friendly relations, and social acceptance were important factors in getting people to comply with requests from others. According to Cialdini, indebtedness contributed to adaptive behavior in primitive societies. He writes:

> Make no mistake, human societies derive a truly significant competitive advantage from the reciprocity rule and, consequently, they make sure their members are trained to comply with and believe in it. Each of us has been taught to live up to the rule, and each of us knows the social sanctions and derision applied to anyone who violates it. Because there is a general distaste for those who take and make no effort to give in return, we will often go to great lengths to avoid being considered a moocher, ingrate, or welsher. It is to those lengths that we will often be taken and, in the process, be 'taken' by individuals who stand to gain from our indebtedness.[15]

Indebtedness is enhanced when the gift-giver is someone we like, but even small gifts from uninvited salesmen or unlikable acquaintances increase the likelihood that we will comply with a request. Many people, after receiving uninvited personalized return address labels in the mail from the American Heart Association, or the National Foundation for Cancer Research, or a nice, free, pocket photo album from Mothers Against Drunk Driving, feel an obligation to make a contribution, and often make one. Even gifts that we discard shortly after they are given can produce an obligation. Why are we so susceptible to such pressures? Presumably because we have accepted and internalized the societal need for reciprocity, we find it unpleasant to be beholden to someone, to be in a chronic state of indebtedness. For these reasons, gifts and favors are powerful influences on us.

The gift of food seems to induce a unique obligation for a reciprocal action, perhaps because satisfying hunger is such a primal instinct. In a clever experiment, researchers at the Center for Hospitality Research at Cornell University engaged servers at an upscale Italian-American restaurant to randomly offer their customers (at the end of the meal) no candy, one piece of candy per person, two pieces of candy per person, or one piece followed by a "spontaneous" offer of a second piece. They then recorded the size of the customers' tips. The tips as a percentage of the bill were (respectively) 19 percent, 19.6 percent, 21.6 percent and 23 percent. The authors "suggest that the more generous the server appeared to be toward the dining party, the more likely she was reciprocated with a greater tip percent. . . . The explanation that appears to be the most plausible in explaining the candy's effect is the norm of reciprocity."[16]

Relations certainly exist between the value of gifts and the tendency to reciprocate. As noted before, even small gifts such as pens and coffee cups produce some indebtedness. And the effect can be long lasting. One of my colleagues, an editor at the *New England Journal of Medicine*, told me that he remembered the pharmaceutical company that gave him a doctor's bag at his graduation from medical school 20 years earlier (it was Eli Lilly)! Larger gifts—substantial fees for serving on a company's advisory board, for example—almost certainly increase the need for reciprocity. There is little doubt that gifts, including free CME and the accoutrements that accompany it, establish a relationship between doctors and industry that obligates the doctor to reciprocate. Although many physicians' self-images protect them to some extent from sacrificing their self-esteem for minor gifts, free CME courses are several orders of magnitude in expense from pens and coffee cups, and the potential influences on physicians are subtler and better hidden. Dr. Stephen Goldfinger, former head of the continuing education department at Harvard Medical School and an early champion of avoiding pharmaceutical largesse, once described reciprocity colorfully. Though his analogy is a bit dated, it captures the context. He wrote, "Indeed, isn't it a bit sleazy to take the corsage without at least yielding its sender a place on one's dance card?"[17]

Too Much Self-Interest

Self-interest is a deeply ingrained, well-hidden human attribute that is strongly tempered by social norms. In the case of physicians, the principal social norms are professional expectations; in particular the notion of putting the patient first and doing no harm. The extreme of self-interest, of course, is greed, implying a desire for more wealth or prestige than one actually needs. Most of the time society channels this tendency into constructive purposes, but sometimes greed triumphs over service to others. Could greed influence some physicians? Could avarice or arrogance (or both) play a role in some of the reactions described before to criticisms of gift receiving? Underappreciation by society—inadequate respect and gratitude for the work—is probably a new influence. The low pay, awful hours, and high stresses during house-staff training probably provide a special stimulus for "payback." These special characteristics may make some physicians more willing to accept drug company largesse as a part of their professional reimbursement.

Denial and Self-Deception

The "self-deceivers," among physicians deserve special attention. How should we take physicians' claims that they can accept gifts without being bought? I am willing to concede that some cannot be manipulated, yet many can, if only at a subconscious level. From work in the field of cognition, we know that introspection and self-reflection are frequently unreliable approaches to appreciating the nature of our thought processes. Human beings often have difficulty understanding or accepting our own motivations; we just can't

easily step outside of ourselves and see ourselves as others do. Human nature is such that people want to preserve their own self-image as honest,
forthright, moral, and ethical people. In particular, physicians see themselves as the prototypical professionals, and as such they believe that others
should simply trust their judgments. As medical students become integrated
into the profession, they develop a self-image that they, too, are moral individuals who cannot be bought.

Physicians know that pharmaceutical companies don't provide these services simply out of altruistic motives, yet they are eager to believe that they
can preserve their integrity in the face of such bribes. How then, do they
cope with the gross discrepancies between the knowledge that they are being
bought and their need to believe that they cannot be bought? Disavowal probably explains much of the mechanism of self-deception. Whereas avowal is a
capacity to identify one's true thoughts and motives, disavowal aids self-
deception by evading these motives. Seen in this light, self-deception is an
unconscious defensive strategy that allows an individual to avoid the pain
and anxiety that accrues with honest avowal of one's actual motives. Disavowal
undoubtedly requires "great persistence and strenuous effort," requiring that
the individual refuse to admit the motive, deny that the motive exists, deny
that there may be negative consequences, and even deny that the motive has
been disavowed.[18] The self-deceiver, of course, often deceives only himself.

This point is illustrated by a small but interesting experiment at the
University of California-San Francisco Medical School. A confidential survey of more than 100 interns and residents sought to determine whether
promotional efforts by drug companies were appropriate and whether the
residents believed that such gifts would influence their prescribing. They
found that the house officers generally were positive about such gifts and
believed that they were uninfluenced by them. Although only 39 percent of
the house officers thought that such pharmaceutical promotions influenced their own prescribing habits, 84 percent thought that the promotions did affect the prescribing habits of others.[19] Moreover, the house
officers' behavior was often inconsistent with their attitudes: not one of the
31 participants who thought that accepting minor gifts (including lunches
at conferences and company pens) was inappropriate had abstained from
accepting them.

Greed has a funny way of working: it is human nature to attribute negative traits to others and to protect oneself, or even to think that one's own ideas rise above all others. Such "cognitive dissonance" has been attributed to dictators who, in suppressing their people and political opponents, assert that they are doing so for the benefit of their society, but it may well apply to anyone with a strong ego who is in a powerful position. In a letter to Thomas Jefferson, John Adams once remarked "Power always thinks it has a great soul and vast views beyond the comprehension of the weak."[20] Some people probably genuinely believe that their acceptance of money from industry yields a benefit not only to them but to society as a whole; others may be aware that their personal gain is uppermost.

Of course, it is simplistic to believe that physicians are uniformly influenced by gifts. Can we avoid being manipulated by the reciprocity rule? Can its attraction be diffused? Cialdini suggests that when we accept a gift we should apply criteria to determine whether the gift was designed to be exploitative. He suggests that, "if the initial favor turns out to be a device, a trick, an artifice designed specifically to stimulate our compliance with a larger return favor, that is a different story. Our partner is not a benefactor but a profiteer; and it is here that we should respond to the action on precisely those terms. . . . As long as we perceive and define the action as a compliance device instead of a favor, the giver no longer has the reciprocation rule as an ally. The rule says that favors are to be met with favors; it does not require that tricks be met with favors."[21]

The idea is that if we believe an attempt is being made simply to manipulate or exploit us, we should redefine the offered gift as a compliance tactic and thus get released from the rule of reciprocity. This idea may be logical, but implementing it sounds like a tricky exercise that could easily be confounded by personal deception. Because of this I do not recommend accepting gifts under any circumstances.

Why Is This Issue So Sensitive?

Discussions of financial conflict of interest induce lively debates and often generate heated emotions. Conflict of interest is a "loaded concept," one with a moral dimension.[22] In some respects it is analogous to other debates with a moral overtone such as when life begins in the fetus, the appropriateness of same-sex marriages, and whether "guns kill people or people kill people." In essence, conflict of interest is a moral stigmatizer: if you choose to have one, it is difficult, if not impossible, to escape the stigma. In addition, people simply do not like to talk about their personal finances: most are too embarrassed to do so.

In many, conflicts create anguish. A young assistant professor told me that he had been struggling with conflict-of-interest issues for three years. After he published several papers describing his research on a certain class of drugs, pharmaceutical companies began offering him grant support for his work and opportunities to consult and give talks for them. He said, "there's all this money flying around," and he wasn't sure how to deal with it. He told me, "I feel that I am working in the gray zone, and sometimes wonder whether I am on the slippery slope—I hope not."[23]

A young trainee at a university hospital discovered quite by surprise that the support of his fellowship did not come from the department, but from a single drug company, and he was repeatedly humiliated when he became known as the LeucoTrial fellow (a fictitious company name). Rather than following his own research interests, he was forced to embark on a clinical trial of the company's newest drug. He was so frightened of retribution that he refused to allow me to use his exact words describing his emotions, even if I changed the quote so that he could not be identified.

A major academic kidney specialist was approached by a company to become a consultant and to testify on its behalf about a drug he had studied to the FDA in the drug's approval process. With angst, he wrestled with the decision either to accept $50,000 for a six-month period, or not to participate. He would like the money, he said, but he worried that any time he would speak about drugs for hypertension and mention the drug, he would be considered "on the take," and his opinion would be discounted. He later he told me that he had decided to be "clean," that is, not to accept any consulting money from industry.[24]

When trying to evaluate responses to financial conflicts and their consequences, one quickly gets into intangible character and motivational issues in which, as described above, even the participants may have no access to their own mental processes.

Wrenching questions have emerged repeatedly throughout my research. Is the person sincere? Can I rely on his principles? On his character? Is he hiding something? Are his actions based on integrity or hypocrisy? What are his true convictions? Is he true to himself? Does he stand up for his principles? It is easy to see how political or legal solutions to such heavily tainted moral issues are nearly always elusive. If so, then the solution to moral dilemmas must include at least some moral precepts. Just because such solutions are difficult and neglected by the profession is no excuse to abandon them. But that these considerations of conflict of interest are so laden with this moral overlay is the most compelling reason for developing working policies that protect honest physicians from being tainted by the stigma.

"Good Work" and the Reluctant Participant

Some, probably a great deal of physician involvement with drug companies, is based on the ethical necessity to do "good work."[25] Faced with declining reimbursement for patient visits, increasing cost of office help and malpractice insurance, the physician who insists on providing good medical care is in a bind. If he spends too much time with each patient, if he is unwilling to cram too many patients into a tight schedule, if he orders too many tests, he may find himself unable to meet his expenses and still make a reasonable living. On a visit to a community hospital in New England in 2002, a director of medical education explained to me that practice income alone was failing to meet even a minimal economic standard that allowed many generalist physicians to live and practice in the community. In an e-mail message he explained:

> The cost of doing business in this part of ———— County is so high that several of the docs have confided that they have trouble making $100,000 annually in a mature practice. This is not sufficient to support a home and even a modest lifestyle in this area. Therefore, the most "ethical"of the physicians (i.e. those who refuse to see more than 20–25 patients a day) look for other sources of income—nursing home medical directorships, stipends from hospitals, drug company "consulting" and legal case review to name a few. It is these activities that bring their income up to a

livable wage. I know specifically of one outstanding young physician who left our medical staff because the clinical revenue from his practice was too low and he was unable to line up any of these outside revenue streams.

I believe that it is important to emphasize that all of these comments have come from some of our best, most professional and hardest working private physicians. They are all Internal Medicine Boarded and come from major Ivy League university training programs. One of the above physicians was actually on the faculty of a major Ivy medical school for several years. These are physicians who refuse to "bulk up" their primary care practices to 60–80 patients a day (which I have seen elsewhere) in order to generate income and they are also docs known for coming in in the middle of the night to see patients when admitted to the hospital. In other words, these individuals are, in my opinion, some of the best in the practicing community. I think it is tragic to see their growing anger and frustration with the medical profession and to have them of necessity, so vulnerable to the discretionary dollars (and modicum of respect) doled out by the pharmaceutical industry.[26]

This comment emphasizes how intrusive market forces, combined with a strong desire to remain in active practice can drive some of the best and most ethical physicians into the willing arms of drug companies. Many of these physicians are among the most honorable among us, who value medicine's legacy of moral standards and practices, and who want to "do the right thing." Yet, they find it difficult to know how. Many are unwilling to focus exclusively on the bottom line and market share. They say that they did not become doctors to practice shoddy medicine, to skimp on tests, to see a patient every eight minutes. Many of these physicians, who eventually become involved with industry, struggle fervently to remain untarnished and preserve their integrity.

The Subtle Influence of Culture

Acceptance of gifts, dinners, consulting arrangements, appointments to speaker's panels, and other perks of industry must be viewed in social context. As long as colleagues are on the take, there is little or no social cost of going along. It seems perfectly legitimate to accept the invitations yourself, and because money is such a powerful motivator, it can inhibit any attempt to ask whether what you are doing is appropriate in a larger, ethical context.

Barbara Toffler's experience at Arthur Andersen, the recently failed consulting giant, is emblematic of the influence of cultural factors. Toffler was hired by Andersen to set up a consulting practice for business ethics, but in the process of trying to bring business into the company, she found herself violating her own canons. She writes, "despite my self-image as a debunker, my frequent battles with my bosses and an occasional outbreak of 'my way,' I basically went along with the culture. I didn't break any laws or violate any regulations, but I certainly compromised many of my values. Some of that was the money talking, but some of it was the fact that if you hang around a place long enough, you inevitably start to act like most of the people around you." She further explains, "It's not a recent discovery that money can be an aphrodisiac, a destroyer of common sense, and as dismissive of intelligence and compassion as any form of power."[27]

Money Talks

Although many physicians deny that they can be influenced by gifts, meals, and the efforts of drug salesmen, the fact that drug companies spend so much money on marketing is silent testimony to the effectiveness of these enormous expenditures. The industry employs large numbers of intelligent people who make their livelihood from marketing. By contrast, physicians spend little time contemplating these issues. In fact, pharmaceutical companies spend more than 21 billion dollars a year on promoting and marketing their products, of which about 88 percent is directed at physicians (the reminder is spent for "direct-to-consumer advertising").[28] With approximately 600,000 physicians in active practice[29] this amounts to more than $30,000 spent on each physician. Although industry market research data are unavailable, studies of physicians show what common sense predicts, namely that physicians are influenced by all kinds of marketing tactics.

Big business and physicians alike are involved in a massive charade. Representatives of the drug companies claim repeatedly that marketing serves an essential function in the health-care delivery system by helping to educate doctors so they can prescribe drugs more appropriately. At the same time, they press their drug salesmen to push the newest (and usually the most expensive) products, and their surrogate intermediaries, the medical education companies, are advertising their services as "persuasive" education. The pressure on drug salesmen is even greater today as many companies' research pipelines have become far less productive of truly innovative new drugs. And despite the yearly marketing budget of the drug industry that is large enough to buy a $50,000 Lexus for about 420,000 people, or pay for a $10,000 family health insurance policy, for about two million uninsured Americans, most physicians still believe that they cannot be swayed by the slanted information they receive from company-sponsored "educational" activities.

Physicians largely believe that they are above being influenced by the largesse of industry, yet considerable evidence indicates that they are susceptible to gifts, meals, and payments. Much of the motivation for accepting such gifts and the mental mechanisms for dealing with it may not even be a conscious process. Financial conflicts of interest are highly charged emotional issues, yet because of the enormous investment of industry in attempts to influence physicians, the public must demand that the profession deal with them more effectively.

YOUR DOCTOR'S TAINTED INFORMATION

IN 1998 HENRY STELFOX AND HIS COLLEAGUES at the University of Toronto rang an alarm. They examined 70 articles about calcium-channel antagonists (including Norvasc, Plendil, Cardene, and Cardizem), drugs that are used for high blood pressure and angina. Stelfox and his colleagues classified the articles according to whether they were favorably disposed toward the class of drugs, neutral about them, or negative about them. They did this in a "blind fashion," that is, not knowing anything about the authors' financial arrangements. They then contacted the authors of the articles and asked them whether they had financial interactions with a number of drug companies that made products for hypertension or angina. Surprisingly, almost all of the authors of these papers returned the questionnaire and checked off whether they had used drug company money to travel to a medical symposium, whether they received an honorarium from a drug company to speak at a symposium, whether they had used drug company money to develop an educational program, or whether they received any money to support their research. Dr. Stelfox's report was illuminating.[1] It said there was "a strong association between authors' published positions on the safety of calcium-channel antagonists and their financial relationships with pharmaceutical manufacturers." They discovered that almost all of the authors (96 percent) who had written favorably about the drugs had financial arrangements with the makers of the drugs. About two-thirds of those whose writing was neutral had such arrangements, and only 37 percent of those who were negative about the class of drugs had financial connections to industry. The report concludes as follows, "We wonder how the public would interpret the debate over calcium-channel antagonists if it knew that most of the authors participating in the debate had undisclosed financial ties with pharmaceutical manufacturers."

Dr. Stelfox and many others think that authors who express their opinions about a test or treatment in a public forum or in writing should disclose financial conflicts they have with any company about whose products they are writing. Yet, disclosure of financial arrangements does not prevent bias; it only alerts a reader that bias might exist.

Dr. Richard Smith, the editor in chief of the *British Medical Journal*, in commenting on Dr. Stelfox's study, went on to cite other examples.[2] He said "The major determinant of whether reviews of passive smoking concluded it was harmful was whether the authors had financial ties with tobacco manufacturers. In the disputed topic of whether third-generation contraceptive pills cause an increase in thromboembolic disease [serious clots in blood vessels], studies funded by the pharmaceutical industry find that they don't, and studies funded by public money find that they do."

These findings merely added to a long-standing concern about bias in the medical literature. Financial conflicts of interest can taint medical information and lead to excessive costs and inappropriate medical decisions. Many people are unaware of the nature of medical information and how their doctors get it.

Your Doctor's Information

Medical information evolves slowly. It comes to light first in medical meetings and then is published in the medical journals. Even though the results of the latest study reported in a journal are often trumpeted loudly in the media, doctors rarely change their practices on the basis of a single study. Medical information is cumulative. A single study appears in a medical journal such as *JAMA* or the *New England Journal of Medicine* only after a rigorous process in which the journal's editors and other experts selected by the editors scrutinize its methods, results, and conclusions, a process known as peer review.

Three or four decades ago, experiential collections of cases treated one way or another were the dominant form of medical information. Typically, a well-known physician treated 50, 100, or 200 patients in his own practice and published his results. When the new results seemed to improve on the then-current approach to treatment, many physicians changed their practices to reflect the advance. Take surgical techniques, for example. When the respected Mayo brothers in Rochester, Minnesota, published their results of a series of abdominal surgical cases, their techniques became the accepted approaches of the day. Despite such reports, however, medical practices often changed slowly, and in some instances not at all. Like politics, medical practices were often a function of local personalities. Physicians who were respected locally for their training, skill, and reputation frequently dominated local modes of practice, even when the practices were not optimal by higher standards elsewhere. Slowly thereafter, the basis of medical practice began to become more scientific. In the mid-to-late 1970s, scientists began to carry out clinical trials that were far more reliable than simple case series. These early studies led to the modern randomized, controlled clinical trial in which narrow clinical questions could be asked by selecting patients to receive either one treatment or another by random allocation, and often blinding those observing the consequences of treatments to avoid prejudicing the results. At first, the National Institutes of Health funded most clinical trials, but in recent years the pharmaceutical industry's support has exceeded that from the NIH.

Regrettably, the improvement in the quality of clinical research was not always paralleled by widespread adoption of the medical advances discovered in the clinical trials. In part, this sluggishness in acceptance of new information is a function of the natural conservatism of doctors, who are taught to be cautious in changing diagnostic and therapeutic approaches to which they have become accustomed, and first and foremost, to do no harm. But conservatism is not the only explanation; doctors had become busier, were reading less, were relying on word of mouth for application of new medical advances, and on "curbside consultations" with local experts for advice about patients' problems outside their immediate field of interest.

Dr. John Wennberg's observations that date from the 1970s were a bombshell. He discovered that there were large variations in the use of some procedures from one community to another. He found, for example, that in Vermont the rate of tonsillectomy in children varied from one community to another between 8 percent to 70 percent. The rate of hysterectomy in women who reached age 70 in two areas not far apart in Maine was 20 percent in one and 70 percent in the other.[3] Even today he finds wide variations in the use of procedures such as tonsillectomy, hysterectomy, and prostatectomy, all procedures for which there is considerable professional disagreement about their necessity. However, for procedures such as appendectomy and hernia repair (for which there is considerable scientific agreement), there is little variation from one site to another.[4]

Wennberg's findings raised serious questions about the consistency of the medical care being delivered across the country, and may have some bearing on why some physicians do more or less surgery for the same condition. One outcome of Wennberg's observations were new approaches designed to improve the quality of care, to identify optimal medical practices, and to introduce some uniformity into what appeared to be—at least for some procedures—more of a crap shoot.

Two of the major efforts to rationalize and codify medical care today are "evidence-based medicine" and "clinical practice guidelines." Evidence-based medicine, a systematic method to combine and summarize the results of controlled trials, involves establishing rigorous inclusive criteria for all published (and sometimes unpublished) clinical trials of a particular treatment (such as the treatment of pneumonia), finding similar patients across the trials, and summarizing the results of their treatment. If rigorous criteria are selected at the outset for including or excluding cases, the recommendations of these evidence-based medicine groups are widely considered to be objective and as a result, physicians can rely heavily on their conclusions.

The second approach is called clinical practice guidelines. Using evidence-based medicine as their basis, detailed summaries of medical problems are prepared and doctors use them in the everyday practice of medicine. Some of these clinical practice guidelines are summaries about how to treat a symptom (depression or pain) or a disease (systemic lupus erythematosus or diabetes), how to make a diagnosis (such as a heart attack) or what to do in certain medical emergencies. Nearly all kinds of medical decisions have been translated into such guidelines. Practice-guideline development is sponsored by the NIH, the Public Health Service, and professional organizations such as the American Medical Association and the American Heart Association. From one organization to another, the extent of in-depth analysis of the subject varies, and although standards for developing these guidelines have existed for more than a decade,[5] the quality of individual guidelines is quite uneven.[6] Because few government agencies or foundations fund such efforts, organizations interested in developing guidelines often turn to industry for funding.

Doctors have access to many other sources of medical information. Some invite pharmaceutical representatives into their offices and conferences, and some attend industry-sponsored conferences. Some avidly read free pamphlets and journals sent to them by pharmaceutical companies. By contrast, some read only the journals that come as part of membership in a professional society, and pay their own money to subscribe to sources that are not dependent on pharmaceutical company support, contain no advertising, and are funded entirely by subscription fees. Such venues include the *Medical Letter* and the computer-aided system called *Up-To-Date*. Many physicians pay for their own continuing medical education.

Because medical evidence changes, sometimes rapidly, it is unrealistic to expect that variation in clinical practices will disappear. And though practice guidelines, even those constructed by experts with no axe to grind, are valuable in guiding treatment efforts, they cannot apply to every patient, and we would not want our doctors to become automatons beholden only to a list of dos and don'ts. In fact, we want them to tailor treatment recommendations for us when appropriate. And of course, we want them to know both the benefits and risks of the medications they prescribe for us, and to be alert for the ever-present side effects.

Drugs save lives and reduce suffering. Ten years ago we had no effective treatment for AIDS or migraine headaches. Twenty years ago we had no treatment for multiple sclerosis, we couldn't prevent heart muscle damage after a heart attack, and we couldn't cure stomach ulcers. Thirty years ago we couldn't prevent kidney damage from diabetes, and with few exceptions we treated cancers with disfiguring surgery. As new drugs became available for previously untreatable diseases and for conditions that were resistant to our existing medicines, we embraced them enthusiastically. Penicillin was the first wonder drug. Introduced 60 years ago, it not only cured deadly infections but, except in rare instances, it seemed to have virtually no ill effects. Penicillin may have spoiled us into thinking that all of our new drugs would behave this way: we surely would have drugs that would cure many diseases without harmful side effects. Unfortunately, we quickly learned that there were nearly always two sides to any new drug: one side was its beneficial effect and the other side its drawbacks.

Some of the drawbacks made us think twice about giving a drug. And in some cases we thought initially that the benefits outweighed the risks but only found later that some patients developed serious complications or even died from our new treatments. Many treatments in use today can cause life-threatening side effects. We treat people with irregular heartbeats (a condition called atrial fibrillation) with a drug called Warfarin to keep their blood from forming clots in their heart, but the thinning of the blood sometimes causes them to have serious bleeding. Similarly, we rush people with heart attacks and strokes to the hospital to give them clot-buster drugs, but these drugs too can cause bleeding, sometimes into the brain. In such cases, the treatment can be worse than the disease. I could go on with more examples, because few drugs have penicillin's very high benefits and low risks. What this means is that any decision about the use of a drug has to take its benefits and risks into account, and that any information doctors receive about a drug has to be carefully balanced and objective. It must not only provide facts about the drug's effectiveness but also its safety. And there's the rub. Not all the information that doctors receive about drugs meets the critical criterion of objectivity.

Medical information is complicated enough even when unbiased. Many medical decisions are made under conditions of uncertainty. Even under the best of circumstances, doctors often have to make diagnoses and recommend treatments before they even know definitively what's wrong with the patient. When the evidence strays from objectivity, they are hampered even more.

There are countless examples in which financial considerations appear to have influenced the information that doctors receive. Some of them come in the form of articles in medical journals, some in the form of Web sites and pamphlets sponsored by pharmaceutical companies, and some in continuing medical education lectures by "opinion-leader" physicians with financial ties to companies whose products they are describing. Their efforts help widen the market for new drugs. Financial conflicts of interest increase the fog around medical decision making, sometimes misleading doctors, distracting them from getting objective information and encouraging them to prescribe unapproved, unnecessary, and unnecessarily expensive medications.

The Role of Medical Editors

Editors of medical journals are supposed to serve as gatekeepers: their job is to analyze the validity of the assessments and recommendations that authors of medical publications make about medical information and medical products. Most editors, at least those at the reputable journals, use peer review by outside experts for an independent opinion about the accuracy, originality, and importance of the work. Editors are expected to let readers know when a recommendation for the use of a product is based on hard facts and when it is based on an author's experience or opinion. Given the critical importance of objectivity in judging when to use a drug, which patients might benefit from a drug, and which patients might respond adversely, doctors and their patients count on the scrutiny of the editors and outside experts to reduce the chance of a biased or faulty recommendation.

The work that appears in medical journals is not just a pure culture of medical facts. It is a complex admixture of straight factual reporting, interpretation of the facts, summary articles, and opinion pieces. Through the peer-review process and their own scrutiny, journal editors have a responsibility to strive toward objectivity and to avoid bias. Unfortunately, because of the press of time and the lack of personal expertise, editors sometimes inadvertently publish overtly biased articles. Even the peer-review process doesn't always protect against bias. Reviewers may not be sufficiently expert to detect subtle bias, and given the extent of conflict of interest among experts in certain fields, reviewers themselves may share the same bias as the author. In my experience, reviewers who are asked to excuse themselves from reviewing a manuscript because they have a financial conflict of interest rarely do. As a consequence, biased information that guides patient treatment can creep into the medical literature, and it does.

Some journals make a distinction between scientific articles and review articles. In scientific articles, original data are presented, allowing readers to judge the facts for themselves. In review articles that summarize a topic (a disease or a symptom, for example), the author selects the medical information and provides his interpretation of the facts for the reader. Thus, in review articles (and editorials as well), there is more latitude for an author to select information that he believes is relevant and important. The benefit of having an author unfettered by financial conflicts is evident: a reader does not have to be concerned that money has stood between the author and himself.

Journals that permit authors to write editorials and review articles about subjects in which they have a financial conflict of interest (as the *New England Journal of Medicine* and the *Annals of Internal Medicine* now do), leave doctors in a quandary, often unable to interpret the disclosed information. Three examples, published all around the same time are illustrative. In an editorial in the *New England Journal of Medicine* in June 2003 about improving the overall quality of medical care, the disclosure listed the author, Dr. Earl Steinberg, as "having equity interests in Resolution Health" (actually, he is the president and CEO of the company), but there was no disclosure of Resolution Health's business activities or their possible relation to any recommendations in the editorial.[7] Given the carefully selected language, a reader cannot determine whether Dr. Steinberg's connection to the company might have bearing on the opinions he expressed. In an editorial in the *Annals of Internal Medicine* in July 2003 about treatment of HIV infection with antiretroviral drugs, the disclosure lists the author's consultancies with 14 different companies and grants from nine.[8] Unless readers are intimately familiar with the field and are familiar with the products of these 14 companies, they would find it impossible to assess whether or not financial conflicts exist and whether or not the commentary might be biased. The third example involves the drug Xigris, a very expensive drug used to treat patients with life-threatening infections (a condition called sepsis). Suffice it to say that Xigris has been controversial from the start: although it appeared to be life saving in a small group of the sickest patients with sepsis, many physicians believed that it should be given to a much wider group of patients who were not so desperately ill. Lilly, the manufacturer, with the help of a small cadre of physicians, has heavily promoted the drug. In July 2003, *JAMA* published a clinical study called the OPTIMIST trial,[9] the second of three clinical trials to find that drugs in the same class as Xigris failed to save lives of patients with sepsis. Despite the negative results, in an accompanying editorial, Dr. Derek Angus defends the use of Xigris. Based on a comparison between the costs and effectiveness of this kind of drug, he opined that Xigris is still worth giving despite its expense.[10] Other experts disagree, arguing that drugs of this type need more study before they are used widely.[11] In a disclosure at the end of the editorial, Dr. Angus notes that he "has received consulting fees, and/or grant support from several pharmaceutical companies involved in the evaluation of antisepsis therapies, including Pharmacia and Eli Lilly." As noted before, Eli Lilly happens to make Xigris. I asked an expert intensive-care physician about Dr. Angus' comments. He wrote,

> Derek Angus . . . should not have been selected to write the editorial given his very close ties to Lilly. In the body of the editorial he mentions the favorable cost effectiveness studies for Xigris (one of these is his own study, a study that was funded by Lilly. . . .). The editorial is a great example of the worthlessness of the fine print financial disclosure. At a minimum, it should state that the author not only participated in antisepsis research for Lilly, but specifically was a principal investigator in their studies of Xigris (the clinical trial and the cost-effectiveness study).[12]

Bias can creep into medical articles in a variety of ways. One way is inattention by an editor to the content of a review article (an article that summarizes a field) that is written by an author who has a financial conflict. Here is a salient example in which an editor seems to have allowed an author with an overt conflict of interest free rein:

In 2003 the *Annals of Internal Medicine*, a respected medical journal, published a review article on the diagnosis and treatment of Fabry disease by authors across the country and in France.[13] Fabry disease is a rare condition that most doctors will never encounter in their careers. Because patients with the condition lack a certain enzyme (protein), they accumulate a fatty substance in small blood vessels that interferes with the function of their heart, brain, and kidneys. Some patients develop strokes and many develop kidney failure. Replacing the missing enzyme is the only effective treatment. Two very similar drugs are available for this purpose: Replagal, made by Transkaryotic Therapies, Inc., and Fabrazyme, made by Genzyme Corp. The authors' recommendations for treating the disorder were extremely aggressive. They recommend, for example, that "enzyme replacement therapy be initiated in all patients with Fabry disease even though important questions regarding dosing and long-term benefits still must be addressed with additional research." They recommend treating children, carriers of the disease trait, and patients with permanent kidney damage even though there is no convincing evidence for doing so. In essence, what they suggested is that the indications for the use of this expensive drug should be broadened to include many patients who are not being treated now, even though the evidence is lacking on the benefits of the treatment. Because Fabry disease is so rare, they say, neither the disease nor the treatment has been studied much, and for this reason, the authors' recommendations are based largely on "clinical experience and expertise" (their own).

Here's the rub. The recommendations were made by a nine-person panel that met face-to-face at meetings (paid for by Genzyme) twice and by teleconference once. The two lead authors of the paper, who selected the other seven participants, are consultants for one or both companies that make the replacement enzyme; one of them owns stock in one of the companies and one has a pending patent licensed to the other company. All seven of the other panelists they selected have one or more of the following financial conflicts of interest with the companies: consultancies, grants, and patents, or have received royalties or honoraria. Thus all of the nine authors have financial ties to one or both companies that make the treatment. In a mere 49 words of a seven-page paper they acknowledge that the treatment (available in Europe) costs more than $150,000 per year.

Would a panel of experts who were not aligned with industry have made the same aggressive recommendations? We have no way of knowing, because the editors of the journal chose to publish a paper by authors who appear to have an axe to grind. Could it be that the aggressive recommendations for diagnosis and treatment represent only zealous concern for patients' welfare? Or do the authors' industry connections warp their proposals?

A senior clinical geneticist, who examined this paper for me, considered many aspects biased. He explained that "the authors' treatment recommendations are inappropriate, and that given a similar patient, testing should first confirm the diagnosis of Fabry disease and if testing is positive, the patient should be asked to enroll in a clinical trial of treatment rather than be given an untested drug."

The geneticist commented, "In regard to this particular marketing piece, one must immediately ask—who actually wrote this and who reviewed it for the Annals? Whose opinion is it that the recommendations are 'Expert,' as per title? The authors or the reviewers? And which author needs to refer to his own expertise in the abstract? If this were editorial comment by the reviewers/editors, it would have some objective value. Coming from the authors, it is advertising. . . . It would take a double pair of CVS specs to read the tiny font size of the 'potential' conflicts of interest. Exactly how potential are these conflicts?"[14]

Are Editors Themselves Compromised?

How much, if any, influence do pharmaceutical companies have on the content of medical journals? Do editors' financial conflicts of interest have any influence on what is published and what is not? Most journals do not have the luxury of full-time editorial staffs, and even editors in chief are often only part time. Assembling an editorial board of physicians who are free of financial conflicts of interest is as difficult as identifying unencumbered individuals to write editorials. When one editor in chief asked me, as one of his "consulting editors," to recommend a financial conflict-of-interest policy for his editorial board, he laughed when I proposed that editors who handle manuscripts should have no financial associations with companies whose products are featured. He said that if he adopted such a policy, he would have no editorial board! When I suggested to a major medical society, which sought my opinion about conflicts of interest in the editorial offices of their six journals, that they could make an important ethical statement by insisting that all the editors who made decisions about manuscripts (the editors and associate editors) have no financial conflicts, they demurred.

During my tenure at the *New England Journal of Medicine* and that of my predecessor, we had a simple rule, namely that the editors themselves could have no financial arrangements with industry, including no stocks in companies with medical connections. The influence of conflict of interest in the editorial staffs of other major journals is not public information and has never been adequately explored. Top physicians in a field are usually chosen to be editors, deputy editors, and associate editors, and they are the very ones who are likely to have financial relations with industry. How they handle these conflicts is not widely discussed. Some probably recuse themselves in discussions about manuscripts in which they have a conflict. Some probably do not. The problem is that recusal is not an ideal solution in small, close-knit editorial groups.

There is also little information about any possible influences of the profitability of medical journals (advertising, reprint orders) on journals' editorial content. I am confident that for at least the last quarter of the twentieth century, these commercial influences had no influence on editorial decisions made by the editors of the *New England Journal of Medicine*, but I have no inside information on other journals. Dr. Richard Smith, editor of the *British Medical Journal*, has raised the concern that lucrative advertising and reprint sales can be a corrupting influence.[15] One experience at the *Annals of Internal Medicine* in 1992 sent a chill down the spines of editors and publishers alike. When the (then) editors, Drs. Suzanne and Robert Fletcher, published a study sharply critical of the pharmaceutical industry,[16] pharmaceutical advertising in the journal declined substantially, and remained lower than usual for months thereafter.[17] For editors of many journals whose profit margins are not robust, that experience might lead them to be chary about criticizing the advertisers who support their publications. These issues are worthy of much more study, but whether editors can be forthcoming about the factors that influence them, and whether the editors' personal financial conflicts influence them in judging what to publish will be difficult, if not impossible, to assess.

Examples of editors that were compromised by commercial considerations rarely come to light, but early in 2004, one did. The editor of *Dialysis and Transplantation*, a journal devoted to the treatment of patients with kidney failure, wrote the following note to the author of a paper that questioned the efficacy of erythropoetin, a commonly used drug marketed aggressively by Ortho Biotech and Amgen, "all three of the reviewers who recommended that your editorial be published were nephrologists (some rather prominent). . . . Unfortunately, I have been overruled by our marketing department with regard to publishing the editorial."[18] The author, Dennis Cotter, believing that the rejection by a marketing manager was an ethical lapse, sent me all relevant documents, and I sent an e-mail message to the editor asking what action he had taken when he was advised that he could not publish the editorial. In return, I received a letter from Tom Blackstone, the journal's director of marketing. In the letter, Mr. Blackstone explained his decision, and concluded by saying, "The highly probable end result would be that *Dialysis and Transplantation* would lose readership and circulation. This is a serious marketing concern, as it would be for any publisher."[19]

Though I had doubts about whether the decision not to publish the editorial had an ethical dimension I urged Mr. Cotter "go public," and recommended several journalists that he might contact. Within a week, the *British Medical Journal* published a short piece critical of the publisher's decision,[20] and days later Deborah Carver, the president of the company that publishes *Dialysis and Transplantation*, reversed the marketing director's decision.[21]

I know that at the most prestigious journals, such action by marketing people is unthinkable, but at other journals that rely heavily on advertising revenue, it may well be quite common. This instance is quite different from most rejections, because the editor was so frank with the author about the rationale for rejecting his paper. Under most circumstances, the editor would simply have rejected the paper without explanation.

Free Continuing Medical Education: Is It Impartial?

Physicians rely heavily on continuing medical education to remain current in a medical science that continues to evolve rapidly. A standard joke in medical training holds that 90 percent of what you learn in medical school will be proven wrong in ten years (it's probably closer to five years now)— it's just that you don't know which 90 percent. CME has become a major commercial enterprise. According to Public Citizen, a watchdog organization in Washington, DC, the yearly revenues for commercial CME suppliers are more than 600 million dollars, and it is growing.[22] Approximately three-quarters of the income of these commercial companies is derived from pharmaceutical companies. Doctors still spend their own money on CME to help study for Board examinations and for attendance at medical meetings of Specialty Societies such as the American College of Physicians or the American Gastroenterological Association, but through the commercial suppliers they also get free education at home and at medical meetings.

The Accreditation Council for Continuing Medical Education (ACCME) requires that commercial support must be acknowledged, that no staff or consultants in the interested company can be involved in the development of the CME activities of the provider, and that the faculty or students be debriefed after each session for their perceptions of possible bias. ACCME also requires that faculty disclose "significant" or "substantial" financial relationships between presenters and commercial entities, and that the physician-students must be made aware if any faculty members refuse to disclose their financial relationships. According to Dr. Arnold Relman, a major critic of commercialized CME, the commercial providers (who are largely supported by pharmaceutical companies and device manufacturers) often enlist faculty who were overly friendly to their sponsor's products despite the ACCME standards and regulations. Dr. Relman argues persuasively that these courses often present information that is biased in favor of the companies that funded the courses, that they sometimes provide information that lacks hard scientific facts, and are not even-handed.[23]

Drug companies often claim that they are just helping the public by providing physicians the best information possible. They admit that they might make friends and generate goodwill for their companies in the process, but their primary goal, they claim, is education, not marketing. The truth about their motives, however, is transparent. One provider of medical education, Joe Torre, the chief executive of an advertising agency that owns its own clinical research company, said, "Very often doctors are more influenced by what other doctors say than what pharmaceutical companies have to say. So companies work through medical education companies to have doctors who support their products talk about their products in a favorable way. That's called medical education."[24]

Pharmaceutical companies spend more than one-half billion to several billion dollars on CME.[25] There is little doubt that they would not spend such sums unless they expected a substantial return on their investment. In fact, in the business proposals that medical education companies make to the pharmaceutical industry, pretenses are dropped. One such company promised drug companies "a collaborative process with a provider who shares your expectations."[26] Another (Hill and Knowlton) offered expertise in pharmaceuticals, providers, payers, policy, and patients "to provide tailored and specific communications solutions to our clients' business challenges."[27] Still another creates "educational programs that foster early product acceptance. . . . Programs are designed to gain a higher rate of acceptance at the launch of a new product and to increase return on investment."[28] Still another says, "Medical education is a powerful tool that can deliver your message to key audiences and get those audiences to take action that benefits your product."[29]

In the mid-90s, in an effort to reduce the influence of pharmaceutical companies on the content of the presentations, the FDA tried to rein in the commercial providers of CME, but backers of commercial CME have effectively blocked them from doing so. In fact, in 2000, a United States Court of Appeals curtailed the FDA's oversight of CME on the grounds that their efforts violated free "commercial speech" under the First Amendment to the Constitution.[30] At present, the integrity of industry-sponsored CME remains a contentious issue in what appears to be a never-ending battle between the FDA and representatives of commercial CME providers.

We should be concerned that the massive pharmaceutical support of CME distorts the information that physicians use to select drugs. Implicit is the notion that this bias leads to prescribing patterns inferior to those under CME sponsorship of academic- and medical-society-sponsored continuing education. Only a few studies have examined potential bias in CME. In one carried out in the mid-1980s at Georgetown University, researchers studied the pronouncements of faculty members on calcium-channel blockers during two CME courses given one year apart.[31] Manufacturers of competing drugs sponsored each course. The faculty's remarks were recorded, transcribed, and categorized: how often the sponsor's drug and other calcium-channel blockers were mentioned, and how often positive clinical effects (such as relief of chest pain) and negative clinical effects (such as constipation and dizziness) were mentioned by the faculty. Though a small study, the results are instructive. In the second course, the sponsor's drug was mentioned many more times than similar drugs and in both courses, more positive statements were made about the sponsor's drug than the nonsponsored drug. The authors conclude that "for both courses there appeared to be some bias in favor of the drug company's drug." In another study the same investigators assessed the drug- prescribing patterns of physicians attending three different CME courses, each of which was subsidized by a different drug company.[32] The physician attendees identified the frequency of prescriptions written for the set of drugs prior and six months after the courses. The authors found that the rate of prescribing for the drug of the sponsoring company increased, while prescribing rates for other drugs described in the program changed little. They concluded that the sponsorship of CME courses does appear to influence physicians' behavior in favor of the company's product. Two caveats: first, these studies are not highly reliable (the number of doctors studied was quite small), yet the concern that physicians are strongly and inappropriately influenced by industry-sponsored CME is a rational one. Second, though these studies are 15 years old, there is no reason to think that the dynamic has changed.

Diagnostic Schemes by Conflicted Authors

Uncertainties in diagnosis dog the clinical definitions of a series of clinical conditions involving the esophagus, the stomach, the biliary tree (gall bladder), and the intestines. These vexing conditions bring hundreds of thousands of patients to doctors' offices with complaints such as abdominal pain, bloating, diarrhea, and constipation. Unlike heart attacks, pneumonia, and diabetes, for which objective tests can verify a doctor's diagnosis, no definitive tests are available that help confirm a diagnosis of functional gastrointestinal disease. What that means is that diagnoses of functional gastrointestinal disease are based instead on a constellation of symptoms. Since 1987, groups of gastrointestinal and psychiatric specialists have been codifying this diverse group of conditions and separating them into entities based exclusively on patients' symptoms, not on biological markers. Drugs represent an increasingly popular approach to treatment of these conditions.

Lay people concerned about the lack of medical attention to these conditions formed a health charity, the International Foundation for Functional Gastrointestinal Diseases (IFFGD), which raises funds for research, publishes pamphlets for the public, works with the NIH in educational programs, develops its own international symposia (five so far) and lobbies Congress.[33] More than 90 percent of the IFFGD's income is derived from 18 pharmaceutical companies, and this support grew by more than tenfold between 1997 and 2002.[34] Pharmaceutical companies also supported committees that held meetings in Rome to classify and reclassify the functional disorders.[35] Certain companies, including GlaxoSmithKline, Novartis, and Solvay, supported the Rome meetings, the IFFGD's meetings, and engaged prominent gastroenterologists and psychiatrists as consultants, lecturers, and researchers. Two of these three companies market drugs used for functional gastrointestinal disorders and the third, Solvay, is conducting clinical trials on another. When "Rome committees" meet and when international meetings are held, experts are invited without regard to their financial ties to these companies. They are only required to disclose such ties.[36]

The ties are quite extensive. Of the seven-member coordinating committee for the upcoming Rome III, for example, four have ties to Glaxo-SmithKline or Novartis and three of the four have ties to both. Two also have ties to Solvay. Of the 87 participants of the 2003 International Symposium on Functional Gastrointestinal Disorders, 31 had financial ties with GlaxoSmithKline or Novartis and 12 had financial ties to both. Ten have ties to Solvay. Employees of Novartis, GlaxoSmithKline, and Solvay were participants in the meeting.[37] Thus, the organization developing standards, a health charity that promotes these functional disorders, and physicians deeply involved with the definition and management of these disorders all have ties to companies that make relevant drugs.

I have little doubt that many patients benefit from these attempts to classify and study functional gastrointestinal disorders and from IFFGD's public education efforts. Yet, although an increasing focus on drugs instead of dietary adjustments and counseling for these disorders may be an excellent strategy for pharmaceutical companies, it may not be ideal for patients. Already, Lotronex, a GlaxoSmithKline drug that was prescribed for patients with irritable bowel syndrome as well as for many patients with minor gastrointestinal complaints, was withdrawn from the market by the FDA only nine months after it was approved because of dangerous adverse effects, including life-threatening ischemic colitis in some patients[38] Do some or many of the gastroenterologists and psychiatrists in this field lean toward industry's objectives? It is hard to imagine that they don't. An excerpt from guidelines for people in the field from an editor's column in the *Functional Brain-Gut Newsletter* entitled, "Working in the FGID's, [functional gastrointestinal diseases] and the Benefits and Challenges of Collaboration with Industry," says, "In recent years I have seen much greater efforts to involve the academician in the production of more scientifically based products, developed in a collaborative fashion. This requires a willingness by both parties to negotiate the product design and its execution, while keeping the interests of both parties in mind. Particularly if you are moderating a symposium or other educational program, it may be important for you and the company to work together on the program's objectives and content."[39]

This isolated quote has broad relevance because the author, Dr. Douglas Drossman, is one of the principal architects of the Rome criteria, the senior editor of *Rome II,* a member of the Board of Directors of IFFGD, the head of IFFGD's planning committee for the 5th International Symposium on Functional Gastrointestinal disorders, an associate editor of IFFGD's official publication, *Digestive Health Matters,* and a respected authority on these conditions. Dr. Drossman has financial ties to Novartis, Solvay, and GlaxoSmithKline.[40]

Promotional Efforts by Conflicted Authors

There are several new "educational ventures" that have the appearance of academic activities, but in fact, are "front organizations" that were initiated by industry and have the net effect of promoting specific products. Companies have engaged prominent academic leaders to head these ventures, collect medically relevant educational content, edit it, and make it available to physicians under the avowed purpose of educating them and improving patient care. Yet the companies not only sponsor the front organizations in their entirety, but also have strong financial ties with many, if not most, of the academic physicians they recruit to generate the material. The medical material looks like ordinary medical content for physician education, but in contrast to articles in mainline medical journals, it is not critically peer reviewed by independent experts who have no financial connections to the sponsors. Although much of the material is probably worthwhile, some is probably subtly biased in favor of the sponsor's products and some of it is grossly biased. These front organizations are continuing to pop up as pharmaceutical companies have come to appreciate the potential marketing value of engaging physicians in their marketing activities. A selected few in the lipid field illustrate the scope as well as the extent of financial ties between the sponsors and the willing physician participants.

The *Lipid Letter* is a publication of a two-year-old organization called Emerging Science of Lipid Management (ESLM). The *Letter* and the organization are focused exclusively on management of lipid abnormalities (disturbances in the fats in the blood) and they focus on treatment with lipid-lowering drugs known as statins. ESLM has held seminars for physicians across the country and has issued "calls to action" for prevention and treatment, many dealing with statins. The lead editorial in the October 2002 issue of the *Lipid Letter* by Dr. Antonio Gotto, the dean of Cornell Medical School in New York and Dr. Peter Libby, chief of Cardiovascular Medicine at Brigham and Women's Hospital in Boston and co-chairs of ESLM, "challenge[d] the medical community to consider whether our present criteria for therapy [with statins] are too conservative," meaning that statins should be used much more widely.[41] Both Drs. Libby and Gotto as well as the six "national faculty" listed in the *Lipid Letter* have financial arrangements with Pfizer (consultantships and membership on Pfizer speaker's bureau), and ESLM is completely underwritten by Pfizer. Pfizer, of course, makes Lipitor, the best-selling statin drug. Even though Pfizer was the sole supporter of the *Lipid Letter*, all makers of statins benefit from wider application of these drugs, which the *Lipid Letter* hopes to achieve. Interestingly, all but one of the eight contributors to the *Lipid Letter* have financial relations with one or more of the companies that make statin drugs (Novartis, Pfizer, Merck, and BristolMyersSquibb).[42]

The Web site, Lipids Online, described as an educational resource, provides articles, slides, and continuing education on atherosclerosis. It is supported by an "unrestricted" educational grant from Merck US Human

Health. (In principle, "unrestricted" means that the grant must be used to support the educational venue, but the company is expected to have no input into its content.) Both articles in a version downloaded in December 2002 featured statins for coronary disease. Of the 14 editors listed on the Web page, ten are consultants or on the speaker's bureau for Merck, and many have financial relationships with many other companies that sell statin drugs.[43] Only two declared no financial conflicts of interest. Drs. Libby and Gotto are editors of Lipids Online as well as the *Lipid Letter*. Merck makes two statins: Zocor and Mevacor.

Lipid Management, a brochure from the National Lipid Education Council that focuses on lipids and their lowering with statins, is also supported by an unrestricted educational grant from Pfizer, as is the Council's Web site.[44] Familiar names abound, including Drs. Libby and Gotto. Dr. Gotto, the chairman of the council, and a consultant for Pfizer, reviewed a recent issue of *Lipid Management* "for medical accuracy." Pfizer, ever busy, initiated the National Lipid Education Council (which publishes *Lipid Management*) when they were launching Lipitor and competing against drugs already available from Merck and BristolMyersSquibb. Dr. Libby and his colleagues offered their advice to Pfizer on the new drug's marketing, and they did the same for AstraZeneca when the company launched another new lipid-lowering drug, Crestor. Subsequently, AstraZeneca agreed to fund a large clinical trial on the role of inflammation in arteriosclerosis, one of Dr. Libby's principal interests.

Why is there a need for three (perhaps more) industry-initiated educational media, all by the same authors, all that deal with the treatment of lipid disorders? Why are the authors willing to lend their distinguished names to three brochures and Web sites that promote statin drugs for companies with which they have a financial conflict of interest? Why not just let the impressive science about the statins speak for itself? I explored these questions with Dr. Libby, a colleague, in a long interview. Dr. Libby earnestly believes that measures to prevent heart disease are vastly underutilized and that tens of thousands of lives could be saved if attention was adequately paid to "preventive cardiology." To advance his beliefs, he partners with many different drug companies, even admitting to "using them" to achieve his educational and research agendas. In exchange for his expertise in helping the companies not only in scientific issues, but in their marketing efforts as well, he and his colleagues receive funds that allow them to spread their educational message to thousands of physicians. Dr. Libby believes that despite the drug-company support of these efforts, strict adherence to published guidelines in creating the content of the sites, multiple layers of peer review by experts, and assessment by his audiences preserves the objectivity of these programs. By disclosing all his financial conflicts of interest and by being involved with so many companies, Dr. Libby believes he can maintain his independence, objectivity, and reputation as an opinion leader in his field.[45] The involvement of these high-level academics in such ventures is open to various interpretations. Dr. Libby asserts that they simply exploit a corrupt system in a way that benefits patients. Nonetheless, to me these relationships between the academics and the companies (which may include providing advice about drug marketing) are too close, too collaborative, and too cozy. They generate income for some of the participants and thus induce some obligation to advocate for the company in unseen ways.

Another educational venture, the National Initiative in Sepsis Education (NISE), was founded by Eli Lilly and Company in 2000 to "deliver information on new therapies [for severe sepsis]." Its educational programs are accredited by Vanderbilt University. All "new content" on the December 2002 Web site dealt with information about the use of Lilly's very expensive product, Drotrecogin Alfa (Activated), or Xigris (the cost of one course of treatment is about $7,000).[46] Financial conflicts with physicians are extensive: six of the ten NISE advisory board members have financial conflicts of interest with Lilly, including research grants, consultant arrangements, and appointments on the speaker's bureau, and 26 of the remaining 61 listed "speakers for NISE Certified CME Activities," have various financial ties to Lilly.[47] Can such conflicts exist without influencing objectivity?

Public Pamphlets That Promote Off-Label Drugs

The biotechnology company Amgen, supports the "National Anemia Action Council" (NAAC), a group of 26 academic kidney doctors, rheumatologists, hematologists, oncologists, endocrinologists, and gastroenterologists.

NAAC, another "front organization," produced a new brochure for the public called *Anemia: A Hidden Epidemic*, which reports that anemia is often associated with many chronic diseases and is underrecognized and undertreated.[48] The brochure has chapters on many different diseases for which the Amgen drug, Epoetin, has not been approved by the FDA. Nonetheless, the chapters hint at "preliminary data" suggesting that there might be a deficit of erythropoietin in these various conditions and that "Epoetin has also shown to be of benefit" in treating many of these disorders. The chapter on heart disease for example, describes "preliminary data in a pilot study" involving 22 patients, surely insufficient information to conclude anything about the effectiveness of the drug. Any patient with one of these conditions who reads the brochure and feels tired is quite likely to ask their doctor if Epoetin is "right for them." NAAC's "AnemiaAlert e-mails also subtly promote off-label uses of Epoetin.[49] In short, the 26 academics have lent their names to what appears to be a marketing tool for Amgen. Not surprisingly, some are consultants for Amgen.

Biased Books

In 2002, doctors all over the country received a handy little book the size of a paperback novel entitled, *Quick Consult: Guide to Clinical Trials in Thrombosis Management*. More than half of the 450-page, inch-thick book is a summary of clinical trials in cardiovascular diseases, but most of the front section consists of monographs on the diagnosis and management of blood clots in veins. The book is a thinly veiled advertisement for Lovenox, a special kind of blood thinner (a form of heparin). Treatments with other blood thinners are given short shrift. Aventis Pharmaceuticals, which makes and sells Lovenox, paid the cost of having a for-profit medical-education company produce the book, and the project editor/author is on Aventis' speaker's bureau and reports having received royalties, commissions, and other compensation relating to the sale of textbooks, reprints of articles, and other written material from Pfizer, Genentech, Aventis, Pharmacia, and Bayer. Of the five other authors of the book, only two had no financial conflicts, the others were all receiving money in one form or another from Aventis.[50]

In 2003, the same individuals were giving Aventis-sponsored seminars around the country to raise awareness of an epidemic of thrombotic disorders. One of my research assistants who attended one such seminar in Boston, perceived an "erosion of objectivity" as the day wore on. He commented that speakers exaggerated the value and underplayed the risks of low molecular weight heparin and that the references provided to the attendees were heavily weighted toward the Aventis product, Lovenox. Thus, in publications and in traveling road shows, the same physicians with substantial financial conflicts are educating physicians.[51]

Objectivity in Clinical Practice Guidelines?

Despite the importance of clinical practice guidelines in the way that physicians practice, wide variations exist across organizations with respect to how such guidelines are developed and how bias based on financial conflicts of interest can be minimized. Practice-guideline development is vulnerable to bias if members participating on panels have financial conflicts of interest with the companies whose products they are reviewing. Even if an organization is reviewing existing data—a seemingly straightforward, objective process—the results can be quite subjective, especially when the requirements of practice exceed the available data. In an important study, Dr. Niteesh Choudhry, a Toronto physician working with the same group that studied possible bias in published reports of hypertension drugs, tried to find out whether guidelines produced by major medical organizations were created by financially conflicted physicians. His team selected the 20 most commonly prescribed drugs in his province (Ontario) and made sure to include common medical conditions such as heart failure, asthma, and pneumonia. They then sent a questionnaire to all the authors of 47 practice guidelines, asking them to relate whether they had a financial interaction with a company that manufactured a drug used to treat diseases that were the subject of the guidelines. They asked them to reveal several arrangements, such as whether they had taken money for participation in a drug-company-sponsored symposium, for their research, for consulting, and whether they had equity in the company. One hundred of the 192 authors they tried to contact completed their survey.[52]

Here's what they found. Nearly 90 percent of the physicians admitted that they had some kind of financial relationship with a company whose drugs figured in the guideline they helped write. Only two of the guidelines disclosed anything about the financial arrangements of the physicians involved. Whereas only 7 percent of the guideline participants thought that their own relationships with industry had influenced their treatment recommendations, 19 percent thought that their coauthors' recommendations had been affected by their industry relationships. Dr. Choudhry concludes that formal methods for disclosure of financial conflicts should be implemented, that the arrangements should be made known to users of the guidelines, and that individuals with "significant" conflicts of interest and those with equity interests in a company that could be affected by the guideline outcome should be eliminated from guideline formulation. Because practice guidelines are often used as a "benchmark" against which the quality of care of a physician or group of physicians is assessed, it is essential that they provide unvarnished, objective recommendations. Needless to say, the financial support of the organizations and the individuals who formulate the guidelines could, in principle, affect that ideal objectivity.

The authenticity of medical information is a fundamental requirement for optimal medical practice, yet doctors can get misled when financial connections between physicians and industry warp the information in medical journals, pamphlets, books, and other educational materials. Financial conflicts can even influence the way that physicians categorize, and thus diagnose, common diseases. One result is unnecessary and inappropriate treatments.

6

OUR OBLIGING PROFESSIONAL ORGANIZATIONS

Nᴇᴡ ᴍᴏᴛʜᴇʀs ᴀʀᴇ ʙᴏᴍʙᴀʀᴅᴇᴅ ᴡɪᴛʜ ɪɴ-
formation about breast-feeding. They are told that breast milk contains everything the baby needs for its nutrition, that it protects them against some
infections, and that it forges a special bond between them and the infant.
Most mothers approach breast-feeding with enthusiasm, but some find that
it doesn't always work as smoothly as nature intended. The so-called latch-on
may be incomplete, and the mother may experience breast pain and engorgement, nipple leaks, and uterine cramps. As if the contrary messages of
nature weren't enough, the new mother also receives contrary messages from
the American Academy of Pediatrics (AAP), the 57,000-member, 74-year-
old professional society of pediatricians. While in the hospital, mothers are
given free samples of infant formulas as well as the academy's extremely
useful booklet titled, *New Mother's Guide to Breast-feeding.* Curiously, however,
the cover of the book displays the name and logo of Ross Laboratories, the
company that makes the popular infant formula Similac. The academy offi-
cially supports breast-feeding enthusiastically, so why would they allow a
formula maker to advertise on their booklet? For profit, of course, to the
tune of about half a million dollars.

The AAP's deal with Ross Laboratories is only one example of the complex web of financial conflicts of interest that plague some of our most
respected professional societies. Several years ago, for example, the American Medical Association made a deal with the Sunbeam Corporation to use
the AMA's name on home products such as heating pads and thermometers
in exchange for royalties on each sale. The American Heart Association

certifies products such as canned tuna fish in return for payment from various food companies. The "industry" Web page of the Endocrine Society invites companies to "get complete access to the endocrine marketplace by partnering with the Endocrine Society." It offers "a solid scientific reputation" and "the full range of endocrinologists you want to reach" with 11 different opportunities "to fit your needs."[1] The American Psychiatric Association is paid by industry to interweave pharmaceutical-company-sponsored lectures with nonsponsored lectures at its annual meeting. The two major allergy societies, both of which receive funding from manufacturers of nonsedating antihistamines, sent a representative to the FDA to prevent less-sedating new antihistamines from being sold without a prescription, thus helping to preserve the profits of the pharmaceutical companies producing these drugs. These are but a few of many examples of the complex ties between professional organizations and industry.

Hundreds of professional organizations represent physicians in every conceivable specialty, subspecialty, and sub-subspecialty. Many, such as the American Medical Association, the American Academy of Pediatrics, the American College of Physicians, and the American Heart Association (AHA) have largely devoted their energies to educational programs, the health of the public, lobbying efforts on behalf of their programs and their members, and support of medical research. (in the last ten years, for example, the AHA funded more than one billion dollars in research grants).[2] In the past, others such as the American Society of Hematology and the Endocrine Society, have had a predominant scholarly focus, with their meetings and journals devoted largely to reporting on the latest research. Yet in many, a narrow scholarly focus is being replaced by increasing involvement with industry.

A brief word about funding from industry. Professional organizations reach out to their members and, more recently, to the public, to alert them about new approaches to diseases of interest. Needless to say, drug companies are as interested in many of the same diseases and treatments as are the professional organizations. In fact, many professional organizations use money donated by industry to support scholarships for young physicians and travel funds for many who would otherwise be unable to attend meetings. Many of these scholarships come with no strings attached and thus allow young physicians to attend meetings when they would be otherwise be excluded because of the cost.

Many publications, Web sites, and programs of the meetings of professional organizations contain the phrase "supported by an unrestricted grant from company X." What does "unrestricted" really mean? When companies first started giving small sums to professional organizations for educational purposes, the moneys were unencumbered and bought little except a bit of goodwill. But these small sums (a $500 or $1,000 grant, for example, to entice a well-known speaker) have been superceded by huge amounts of money offered by multiple companies. Although the pharmaceutical companies are not particularly interested in offering money to support professional societies' operating expenses, many professional organizations depend on them to do so. Many believe there is frequently some quid pro quo, namely, a desire of the drug company to leverage its gifts to foster its marketing efforts. Thus, the companies often support specific projects, some initiated by the professional organization and some by the company, that involve one of their products. In addition, they may offer logistical support such as ghostwriters who pen materials for busy physicians, and they are permitted to recommend speakers for meetings and authors of practice guidelines who are sympathetic to the company's marketing objectives, even authors who are paid consultants to their company. Although the organization need not accept a company's choice of topic or authors, when they do not, future funding may be in jeopardy, especially at a time when dues from members are declining. Even a proposed project may never see the light of day if the company perceives that its best interests are not being served. One doesn't have to be an economist to appreciate that the drug companies have a vested interest in supporting these kinds of professional society efforts, and that they are almost certainly not doing so only out of the kindness of their hearts.

Professional societies, often in jeopardy of losing members as dues rise, or intent on continuing to grow their programs, are susceptible to offers of "unrestricted grants." Many who accept unrestricted grants try hard to "keep on message," namely to produce as unbiased material as they can. Some succeed. Some do not. It is easy to see why they do not, when you examine the amounts of financial support and the breadth of it. A few examples from the Center for Science in the Public Interest:[3]

In 2002 the American College of Cardiology gave Pfizer their Diamond Heart Award for a donation of $750,000, AstraZeneca and Merck received the Platinum Heart Award for more than $500,000, and Aventis, Bristol-Myers Squibb, GlaxoSmithKline, and Proctor & Gamble Pharmaceuticals got the Gold Heart Award for more than $250,000. Six more drug and device companies received the Silver Heart Award for donations greater than $100,000. Half of the remaining 28 donors who gave more than $10,000 were drug or device companies. Twenty-four of 26 of the American Academy of Family Physicians' top "corporate partners" are pharmaceutical companies. Top givers ($40,000 or more) are AstraZeneca, Bristol-Myers Squibb, Eli Lilly, Purdue Pharma, and Schering. The American Academy of Neurology lists 75 "corporate donors." Many are drug companies. Nearly all of 30 corporate sponsors of the American Society of Clinical Oncology (only a partial list) are pharmaceutical or biotechnology companies. The American Academy of Orthopaedic Surgeons' Corporate advisory Council is open to any orthopaedic-related company that pays yearly dues of at least $1,000. In 2003, 41 companies were members.[4] Needless to say, this list is incomplete. Similar readily available public records of most professional organizations do not exist.

We must consider the consequences of these ever-increasing financial entanglements between our medical associations and industry. Are medical organizations' objectivity in scientific and medical matters threatened by these collaborations? How much of their oft-stated goals to serve the public first are empty rhetoric?

The Cardiologists

Cardiology is a perfect setup for financial conflicts of interest. Cardiologists deal with life-threatening conditions that are amenable not only to preventive methods (with drugs) but to emergent treatments with expensive drugs and technology, which in turn are the focus of aggressive marketing efforts by industry. In addition, cardiologists take care of millions of patients with these conditions every year, so the market for the drugs they use is huge. Backing them up are two impressive organizations, the American Heart Association and the American College of Cardiology (ACC), each with tens of thousands of members. People often encounter the widely recognizable AHA red heart containing a checkmark at restaurants, denoting AHA-approved foods and menu items. The annual meetings of the AHA and ACC are attended by many thousands of people from all around the world. Pharmaceutical company representation at these meetings is not only impressive, it is overwhelming. The cardiology organizations are, I believe, still learning the complexities of dealing with conflict of interest.

As do many other professional organizations, the AHA and ACC develop clinical practice guidelines for doctors. In fact, the two organizations cooperate to develop and publish some joint guidelines, thus giving the powerful imprimatur of both organizations; they have produced more than a dozen since 1995, and some early ones have undergone revision. The process by which these organizations develop guidelines has been finely honed and firmly institutionalized. Leaders in cardiology believe that this process insures that recommendations are supported by all available evidence, yet suspicions have been raised over the years that some of their guidelines have been influenced by their connections with industry. As a result, the American Heart Association has lost some credibility. This compromise in the integrity of its reputation may not be deserved, but it is easy to see how it occurred. Given the criticism, it is worth exploring how the AHA's guideline process works. Officers and a chair of an ongoing clinical-practice-guideline committee of the AHA have been open and forthcoming in conversations with me about their procedures.

When a new guideline is planned, a joint committee of the AHA and ACC recommends physicians to chair the committee, and together the presidents of both organizations make the selection. The chair then solicits recommendations for participants in the writing committee from a variety of organizations (The American College of Emergency Medicine, for example) and then passes his proposed slate to the joint committee for approval. All possible participants for the writing committee have identified their financial conflicts of interest (by the honor system), and the joint committee has this information when it makes its selections. Although nobody has been dropped from a writing committee because of a conflict of interest, AHA officials told me that some people are not appointed when their conflicts of interest are deemed too extreme. (There are no set criteria for what might constitute "too extreme.") At the beginning of each meeting of the writing committee, each member states the name of the company or companies with which he has a financial arrangement.[5] Participants are asked to voluntarily excuse themselves when one of the companies could profit from their participation.[6]

Nonetheless, nobody monitors whether this requirement of abstention is regularly implemented. In addition, the conflicts of interest of writing committee members have never been published, though the next guideline for a particular type of heart attack will contain the financial conflicts of all participants.[7]

The guideline process is not impervious to influence. Because committees typically consider a formal "evidence-based" review of all possible evidence too tedious and expensive, they instead base much of their analysis on the combined knowledge and wisdom of the members of the guidelines committee (which can be quite extensive). As a consequence, the process can be vulnerable to various influences, both internal and external. Individuals with strong personalities and strong opinions, and even strong agendas, can dominate the process. Pharmaceutical company employees who learn about the inner workings of the committee can try to influence individual members in how their drugs are rated. Even if a professional organization involved in guideline development wanted to hold its panel members to strict confidentiality, it would be difficult to do. By its very nature, guideline development requires wide consultation and discussion with many experts, not all of whom can be on the committee.

All diagnostic tests and drugs given to patients are evaluated according to the same scale. Class 1 is reserved for drugs, tests, or treatments for which evidence or general agreement exists that the treatment is beneficial and effective; Class 2 consists of treatments for which the evidence is either conflicting or opinion is divergent about efficacy, and Class 3 consists of treatments for which evidence or expert opinion indicates no efficacy or even harm. Needless to say, disagreements often exist about the category in which a given drug is placed. Some drugs that have a beneficial effect in the tightly controlled environment of a multicenter clinical trial, for example, may not work as effectively in local communities, where teams of physicians may be less well coordinated to provide care or where drug administration may not be as reliable. In addition, bias in favor of one or more drug companies could also inflate the rating of a drug or class of drugs.

No matter what the explanation for disagreements, differences of only one category can have profound implications because pharmaceutical companies intensively market their new products depending on these guidelines. Some even heavily promote a product if it gets anything higher than the lowest recommendation. After the 2000 AHA guidelines for cardiopulmonary resuscitation gave the Wyeth drug, Amiodarone, a "possibly effective" rating, for example, the company marketed the drug aggressively.[8] The company cited that it was the only drug recommended for emergency treatment of the condition by the AHA!

The use of the drug Alteplase for stroke is a perfect example of how financial arrangements between a professional organization can taint a clinical guideline. Until recently, neurologists had little to offer a patient who suddenly became paralyzed with a stroke. Much of the time the paralysis is permanent and seriously disables the sufferer. Based on the success of clotbuster drugs such as Alteplase in opening coronary arteries and reducing the injury to heart muscle when the drug is administered rapidly to patients having a heart attack, the NIH initiated a study of Alteplase to see if the drug could save brain tissue in patients suffering strokes. Strokes, like heart attacks, require quick action to prevent the damage of brain tissue. But with strokes there is an added problem: because bleeding into the brain, rather than clots in the arteries, causes some strokes, giving Alteplase (which dissolves clots and also prevents them from forming) to bleeding patients can be catastrophic. It can worsen the stroke and increase the chance of death. Thus, in addition to acting as soon as possible, a diagnostic test has to be done within minutes of the start of symptoms to show whether a clot in a brain artery is the cause of the stroke.

The initial studies of Alteplase were encouraging. In many patients brain tissue appeared to be rescued, significantly lessening the paralyzing effects of the strokes on suffers.[9] At last neurologists had a treatment that would sometimes reverse the terrible effects of clotted arteries to the brain! True, some patients developed bleeding in other sites and some died of bleeding, yet the overall benefit seemed to outweigh the risk. Stroke teams were established at many hospitals to deal with "brain attacks," as the American

Stroke Association described them to the public, which had long understood the condition "heart attack." The American Stroke Association, a
branch of the AHA, set about to inform the public about strokes, including
the need for immediate hospitalization of anyone whose symptoms suggested that a stroke was coming on.

But not all physicians agreed that the benefits of giving Alteplase for
acute strokes outweighed the risks. A prominent critic, Dr. Jerome Hoffman,
a clinical epidemiologist at UCLA, was on the AHA guideline panel in 1998
on the treatment of stroke and wrote a minority report offering a dissenting interpretation of the evidence. Hoffman's interpretation, which is shared
by many physicians and more than one emergency medicine professional
organization, is that the Class 1 recommendation for the use of Alteplase
was based on only a single (though well-performed) clinical trial[10] and that
other less tightly controlled clinical trials showed negative effects.[11] He also
argued that the risk of bleeding outweighs any benefits of Alteplase when
the drug is not used as precisely as it was in the highly organized and rigidly
controlled structure of the clinical trial. Other analyses of community-based
patients, including one in Connecticut by a group at Yale University, supported this view.[12]

When the 2000 AHA Guidelines gave Alteplase the Class 1 recommendation, Hoffman's dissenting report was not published, and his name was
even expunged from the list of participants. The differences of opinion
soon spilled over into the public arena. Jeanne Lenzer, an enterprising
freelance medical journalist, published a piece in the *British Medical Journal*
laying out some of the scientific arguments, but claiming that one of the
possible reasons for the Guideline's preference for Alteplase treatment was
a major financial association between the AHA and Genentech, the manufacturers of the drug. Lenzer pointed out that the AHA had received 11
million dollars from Genentech in the prior ten years, and that six of the
eight guideline panelists had ties to Genentech or its marketing partner,
Boehringer Ingelheim.[13] Lenzer concludes, "This recommendation [the
Class 1 designation for Alteplase in acute stroke] may have been made in a
true spirit of unbiased scientific inquiry, but the appearance of dispassionate analysis was eroded by large donations from a drug company to the

organization making the recommendation and payments for research and lecture fees to its individual expert panelists."[14]

This quote exemplifies the AHA's political problem and the more important problem of the average doctor trying to decide how best to treat strokes. Let us assume that the AHA-Genentech funding connection and the conflict of interest of members of the guideline committee had absolutely no effect on the Class 1 recommendation for Alteplase. In fact, in a letter to the editor of the *British Medical Journal,* the president of the AHA vigorously denied that conflict of interest had influenced that particular recommendation.[15] Still, the major financial connection with the manufacturer of Alteplase has tainted the AHA's reputation. Unfortunately, what began as polite differences of opinion degenerated into allegations of selective use of science, accusations of bias, and name calling. Officials of the AHA dismiss the allegations of bias as fringe arguments, and deny their validity. Yet they have not recovered from what is, at the minimum, a substantial public relations problem, and their procedures for developing guidelines do not protect them from further allegations of bias.

Are the disagreements about AHA guidelines only the result of different interpretations of the same data? Are the leaders who chose the chair and members of the committee unimpeded and unmoved by their personal relations (or their organization's relations) with industry? We would not be asking these questions if the AHA had selected individuals with no financial arrangements with industry, or if they had not relied on huge donations from industry to support their programs.

There are other serious implications for the practice guidelines of professional organizations. Managed-care organizations, hospitals, and other institutions increasingly use such clinical practice guidelines as benchmarks for the quality of care by physicians and groups of physicians, thus directly affecting the way in which patients are treated on a day-to-day basis. Thus, if a Class 1 drug is underutilized for heart attacks by a physician group, the physicians may be penalized or embarrassed for delivering suboptimal care (or possibly even sued for malpractice),[16] even though there may be considerable uncertainty about whether the drug should have been placed in a lower class. This problem also arises when industry supports clinical registries.

Clinical registries compile information on a particular disease or the effect of a particular drug from physicians or institutions around the country (or around the world), summarize the information, and then report their observations. Registries are useful in identifying patterns of disease, side effects of drugs, beginning epidemics, and in clinical research. Cardiology has several, including NRMI, the National Registry of Myocardial Infarction. This registry, now 12 years old, encompasses about 1,600 hospitals and about 1.7 million patients. It tracks high-risk patients with heart attacks, summarizes their findings, and supplies the data it collects to the hospitals in its network. One of the newest registries got started a few years ago when representatives from Millenium Pharmaceuticals and Key Pharmaceuticals offered to fund a registry devoted to acute coronary disease at the Duke Clinical Research Institute.[17] Millenium's perspective, they explained, was that there was a gap between the recommended use of certain anticlotting drugs in the AHA/ACC guidelines for NSTEMI (a certain kind of heart attack) and the drugs' actual use in practice. Such a gap, they said, was indicative of substandard quality of care. Subsequently, several other companies that market drugs used in the treatment of coronary disease also added their financial support to this program. Duke created the registry, developed an impressive, expensive package of brochures to describe it, billed it as a "National Quality Improvement Initiative," and called it CRUSADE.[18] CRUSADE already has data on more than 75,000 patients from more than 500 sites in its database.[19]

In fact, there is a gap between the recommendations of established guidelines and the use of various drugs for NSTEMI, and there is a legitimate role for efforts to close the gap. Clearly, many patients are better off because industry has become involved in these quality-improvement efforts. But whether the pharmaceutical industry should be so deeply involved in such initiatives is open to question. Because registries such as CRUSADE are used as standards against which the performance of physicians and hospitals are assessed, and because industry-supported registries have no obligation to adhere strictly to guidelines such as those of the AHA, it creates a situation rife for abuse. An examination of CRUSADE provides valuable insights. Some of the physicians who manage the registry have personal financial ties (consulting and speaking arrangements) with Millennium and

Key Pharmaceuticals.[20] These companies market Integrilin, an anticlotting agent used intravenously for coronary patients. An inordinate amount of space in the CRUSADE brochure is taken up with discussions of Integrilin and its cousin anticlotting drugs,[21] and the brochure suggests that there is substantial underutilization of these drugs. In a telephone conversation, one of the CRUSADE developers admitted that the brochure was somewhat tilted toward Integrilin.[22]

Although the CRUSADE recommendations are based on the clinical practice guidelines of the AHA and ACC, they do not necessarily adhere to the guidelines precisely. Though the details of the difference between the standards of the AHA/ACC guidelines and the CRUSADE registry are far too arcane for consideration here, suffice it to say that CRUSADE went beyond the guidelines in promoting the use of the anticlotting drugs of its industry sponsors, especially Integrilin. Several cardiologists, including those who helped develop the AHA/ACC guidelines, objected to these CRUSADE standards because they believed that the evidence was insufficient to recommend Integrilin as a quality standard.

Thus it does appear that the industrial connections can influence registry printed materials and accountability standards. Doctors could be much more confident about how to interpret the information about the value of such drugs if registries used for quality improvement were supported by an independent government agency such as the Agency for Healthcare Research and Quality. Should pharmaceutical companies be responsible for "national quality initiatives?" Clearly it's good for their business; maybe it should be none of their business.

The Allergists

In the past, people with hay fever suffered from itchy eyes and runny noses or from the side effects of the antihistamines used to treat their symptoms. The discovery of the new antihistamines Allegra, Claritin, and Zyrtec offered these patients great relief. After many years on the market, the safety of the new drugs was assured, so much so that some advertisements for them claimed that they had the same side effects as sugar pills. For many years the new antihistamines were available without a doctor's prescription ("over-the-counter") in other countries, including Canada, a country with particularly stringent drug regulations.[23] But they were not available over the counter in the United States.

The medical insurance industry, led by Wellpoint in California, was eager for the FDA to allow their customers to purchase the new nonsedating antihistamines over the counter. They had everything to gain by such an action because prescription drug coverage (when you have it) rarely pays for nonprescription medications, and thus the insurers would no longer be required to cover the cost of these drugs.[24] Of course, patients would have to pay out of their pockets instead. Nonetheless, over the long run, moving these drugs to over-the-counter status wasn't a bad idea. Although the drugs were quite expensive at the time, they were already cheaper in other countries, and once the drug faced competition with others, there was a reasonable expectation that its price would fall.[25] Because the new drugs were quite safe if they could be bought at any drug store, patients could get the drugs when they needed them without the bothersome step of trying to reach their doctors or return for unneeded office visits. Initially, the three drug companies that make and market the drugs, Aventis (Allegra), Schering (Claritin), and Pfizer (Zyrtec), were opposed to the change in status.[26]

The FDA, which approves such changes, put together an advisory panel in May 2001 to look at the proposal. The two major professional allergy societies, the American Academy of Allergy, Asthma, and Immunology (AAAAI), and the American College of Allergy, Asthma, and Immunology (ACAAI), sent a joint representative, Dr. Bobby Q. Lanier to the meeting. Lanier was then president of the ACAAI, a member of its Government Relations Committee, and the past president of the County Medical Society of the Fort Worth, Texas area. To judge by his awards, he was widely respected in the AMA and in the allergy societies. To top it off, he is handsome and articulate, in fact, more than the run-of-the-mill allergist: he had served as an NBC television correspondent, founded the National Association of Physician Broadcasters, and is seen or heard daily in 72 television markets and in more than 250 radio stations.[27] The perfect spokesman. Given the interest that individual allergists and their organizations have in improving the quality of life for allergic patients, it would be a reasonable assumption that Dr. Lanier would argue for allowing patients to buy the drugs over the counter.

He didn't. Cost to the patient wasn't the only argument. Instead, he argued that eliminating physicians from the care process would lead to inappropriate drug use, overuse, poorer outcomes, and trivialization of the disorders for which the drugs are taken.[28] He offered little evidence for these opinions, with which many other respected allergists disagree. The counterarguments were straightforward: the drugs, if anything, were safer than those already available over the counter, and no evidence of poorer outcomes had emerged in countries that already allowed free access to the drugs. A former president of the AAAAI, who favored allowing access of the public to the drugs, was met with a deaf ear when he tried to learn why the leaders of the AAAAI and the ACAAI opposed the change.

One speculation was that the allergy societies were simply trying to protect their profession's involvement in the care of allergic patients. But other motives may have been at play, given the complex financial entanglements of these organizations and the pharmaceutical industry. Schering-Plough, the manufacturer of Claritin, was a sponsor of the AAAAI Web site at the time and is a major sponsor of more than a dozen local and national programs.[29] Aventis, the manufacturer of Allegra, was a major financial supporter of the annual meeting of the AAAAI. At the meeting in 2001 in New Orleans, for example, Aventis supported the president's reception and the president's research award, brunches and dinners for trainees, a reception for international attendees, a distinguished lecture series, a membership directory, registration bags, and a kiosk for messages.[30] According to the 2002 Web site, Aventis gave AAAAI a "generous educational grant" to sponsor its speaker's bureau and support some of its research awards as well.[31] AAAAI openly solicits industry support of its national meeting. Its 2002 Web site lists 23 activities totaling more than $700,000, including its registration list ($25,000), Board Dinner ($10,000), child-care services ($15,000), Internet Café ($18,000), and President's Reception ($75,000).[32] What AAAAI gives in return, if anything, is not mentioned.

The allergy societies had overt financial conflicts of interest with the companies who make the nonsedating antihistamines. The companies had much to gain by preventing the drugs from being sold without a prescription, and the allergy societies had much to lose if the drug companies reduced or withdrew their support. Where was the welfare of allergic patients in this complex mix of interwoven alliances? Was the avowed mission of the AAAI to provide "optimal patient care to the over 50 million Americans suffering from some form of allergic disease" being well served?

The Pediatricians

Many members of the American Academy of Pediatrics were dismayed that the Academy had accepted a large payment from Ross Products to affix the Ross name and logo on the official academy book that promoted breast-feeding. The characteristic teddy bear of the company, a division of Abbott Laboratories, adorns the 2002 cover of the "New Mother's Guide to Breast-feeding." This industrial "tattooing" was quite a surprise to many members of the academy because it ran counter to a long-standing academy principle that promotes breast-feeding and discourages the use of commercial formula. When controversy arose about the decision, the academy's executive director, Dr. Joe M. Sanders, admitted that such a deal would have been unacceptable ten years earlier, but that it was now an industry "standard."[33] A spokesperson for the company declared, disingenuously, that they agreed with the academy's position that breast-feeding was the best approach, and that the "company wants to provide the best information possible." There is little doubt, however, that Dr. Sanders understood that Ross had different motives, because he harkened back to his own experience when he accepted medical textbooks from industry. He said, "Obviously the advertising works."[34]

Melody Petersen, the *New York Times* reporter who described this arrangement, estimated that the company had paid more than a million-and-a-half dollars to purchase the breast-feeding book but that Dr. Sanders indicated that the academy's profit amounted to no more than $500,000. She also reported that formula makers were major supporters of the annual budget of the American Academy of Pediatrics.[35]

Many members of the Academy of Pediatrics who helped write the book were incensed, believing that the academy had sold out. Dr. Lawrence Gartner, emeritus professor of pediatrics at the University of Chicago and chair of the AAP Section on Breastfeeding, wrote this to Dr. Sanders on behalf of his section:

This imprint ("Ross Pediatrics" and their product logo) gives the reader of the book the distinct impression that the book was sponsored by an infant formula manufacturer and may contain material, which is favorable to the commercial interests of the company. More specifically, the potential reader may have the unfortunate impression that the book will not contain the full scientific and clinical facts about breast-feeding and lactation that a book from the AAP should contain. In short, it devalues an excellent and important book. We who were involved in the writing and editing of the book know that Ross Laboratories was never involved in any way with the preparation of the book.

Of greater concern to us is the harm that may come to the image of the American Academy of Pediatrics as a strong advocate of bre·st-feeding. . . . many of our members and a large number of non-members will see this as evidence that the Academy has sold itself to the highest bidder at the expense of our breast-feeding effort.

The members of the breast-feeding section then asked that the leadership of the American Academy of Pediatrics develop a strong policy to assure that commercial names, products and logos were never again placed on any educational materials of the Academy.[36] Although a large number of the 800 members of the breast-feeding section apparently agreed with this viewpoint, most pay little attention to these issues.[37]

The response from Dr. Sanders follows:

> . . . providing quality educational and advocacy efforts for both pediatricians and the children they serve is not an inexpensive process. Our . . . membership dues generate less than 25% of the revenue required to meet our expenses. This business arrangement we negotiated with Ross afforded us the opportunity to generate some non-dues revenue.
>
> There has also been some concern expressed by some of the approximately 25 pediatricians we've heard from on this issue that this cover modification will tend to discredit the content of the manual. I personally do not feel either would be the case. . . . I think we should assume that the majority of breast-feeding mothers have the ability to draw their own conclusion, and will not assume that the content of this manual has been developed to support a commercial interest. My conversations with

the corporate leadership at Ross suggest that they view the breast-feeding mother as a "futures market."

The Academy's Board of Directors already addressed this issue [of not allowing commercial names, products and logos] . . . on any educational and promotional materials of the American Academy of Pediatrics] and has supported the reality that it has been and will increasingly be necessary to join in mutually beneficial activities with corporate sponsors.[38]

At first glance this does seem like a "win-win" arrangement. Ross is making it possible for a great many women to get an excellent book. What could be wrong with that? Unfortunately, it's not that simple. Both the company and the medical society are playing transparent games. Leaders of the academy seem to be pretending that branding its product has no influence on new mothers' decisions to breast-feed their infants. Many individual academy members pretend that taking pharmaceutical money has no influence on their organization. Industry pretends that its logo and name are invisible and it is simply supporting a book on breast-feeding out of the goodness of their hearts. Everybody knows what the real motive is: even for those women who might choose to breast-feed, get them to use commercial formula instead.

The Pulmonologists

After its 2002 International Conference, the American Thoracic Society (ATS) published two widely distributed items. The first, a brochure titled, *ATS 2002 Conference Symposia Excerpts,* consists of four sections that cover diverse topics of special interest to lung doctors.[39] A different pharmaceutical company supports each section: in fact, each is supported by a company whose product is mentioned prominently in the corresponding sections. The author of *Symposia Excerpts,* Kurt Ullman, the president of a company called Medical Communications, liberally quotes speakers at the conference, and in each instance he selectively uses speakers' quotes that lend credibility to the assertions, but that strongly promote the use of a drug produced by the company that sponsored the section.

Titles of several sections are misleading: one titled, "Social and Economic Implications of Severe Sepsis" (supported by Eli Lilly and featuring the remarks and a photograph of Dr. Derek Angus) had no social implications and only two sentences about economics. In effect, the publication is more a paid advertisement for industry than a publication of a learned medical society. In fact, the misleading headings are only part of the deception. The title, *Symposia Excerpts,* misleads the reader to thinking that he is reading selected summaries of key talks on the formal schedule of the conference. In fact, they are summaries of after-hours conferences sponsored by pharmaceutical companies. Despite the assertion on the cover that the *Symposia Excerpts* is a publication of the ATS, the ATS carefully disavows responsibility with a disclaimer that reads: "The opinions expressed in this publication are those of the speakers and do not necessarily reflect the opinions or recommendations of their affiliated institutions, the publisher, the American Thoracic Society, or any other persons."[40]

All three of the physicians who I contacted and who were quoted in the *Symposia Excerpts* were dismayed that their remarks had been taken out of context, and that they were made to seem like hawkers of industry products. None said that they had complete control of the text of the publication. One was quick to tell me that he had never owned equity in the company whose drug he had discussed and that he had received less than $1,000 for his participation in the symposium.[41] Another said that he had prepared his talk on his own and had been unaware that his material would appear in the *Symposia Excerpts.* He said, "I share your perception that this post-meeting publication appears to be nothing more than a paid synopsis of the post-graduate programs which were funded by industry."[42]

Boehringer Ingelheim, a pharmaceutical company that makes and sells several important (and very effective) drugs that lung specialists use frequently, was one of the companies that supported the *Symposia Excerpts.* It also paid for the second publication of the 2002 conference, the official newsletter of the ATS.[43] In return, Boehringer Ingelheim not only got their logo on the masthead of the newsletter but a four-page, glossy, color insert in the middle that advertises one of their products. An uninvolved pulmonary specialist described this arrangement as "pretty explicit and disgusting."[44] For its investment, Boehringer Ingelheim also received a direct link from the ATS Web site to its own, and a 500-word description of its products on the ATS Web site.

Thus, the ATS allowed a company to emblazon its logo and products on its official newsletter and it allowed a medical writer to use carefully selected quotes of experts to promote pharmaceutical company products. It all comes down to this: how much is it worth to the ATS to compromise its reputation and to impugn the reputation of its members who give talks at its meetings? The president of the society declined to tell me why the society does not eliminate the *Symposia Excerpts* or to provide me, in response to my e-mail request, details on payments made for sponsored evening symposia or other details of the society's contractual relations with industry.

The Critical Care Doctors

The business practices of the Society of Critical Care Medicine, the main professional organization of physicians who care for the sickest hospitalized patients, are the very embodiment of the kinds of conflicts of interest professional organizations are willing to tolerate. At SCCM's annual meetings, just about everything is for sale. Aside from the usual sponsored meetings in the evenings, a company can even pay hefty sums for the talks given within the meeting. The program lists the talks as sponsored by an educational grant from the company, and the company is allowed to show its logo on the signs that announce the talks. According to a member of the organization who regularly attends the meetings, financial conflict-of-interest disclosures of the faculty do not usually accompany the title of the talk in the program, and to find them it is necessary to search elsewhere.

The Web site for the 32nd meeting of the organization in San Antonio held early in 2003 contained a 20-page insert entitled *Sponsorship Opportunities*. The more than 50 opportunities for sponsorship add up to approximately two million dollars. They included the opening reception (can be purchased by a company for $100,000), the President's Reception ($30,000), the Rustlers Rodeo Roundup ($150,000), the Chili Cook-off ($5,000 each), the Internet Pavilion ($40,000), and various educational grants ($125,000 for the President's Circle, $75,000 for Platinum level, $50,000 for Diamond level, etc.). For various smaller sums, companies can buy tote bags, pens, highlighters, and notepads for all the participants.[45]

Detailed lists of the benefits of sponsorship are given. For an investment of $75,000, for example, a company can obtain the "Plenary Session Package," which lists the plenary sessions as "the highest draw events of the Congress." The brochure lists six topics, each undoubtedly of great interest to one pharmaceutical company or another. If they buy one of these events, they get "Recognition of sponsorship from the podium by the SCCM President during Opening Session," and their logo displayed on the screen whenever a slide is not in use. For a mere $65,000 a company can buy session highlights on CD-ROM. Included in this package is the company's ability to select up to four educational sessions on a single CD-ROM, and the sponsor's logo will appear on the label and all screens. Fifteen thousand dollars buys a sponsor a Relaxation Station, where the buyer can "capture qualified leads as prospects seek out your booth asking for vouchers to redeem for a great massage."[46] An entry on the SCCM Web site entitled "Advertising and Sponsorship Opportunities" reads, "Are you looking for a winning strategy to enhance patient care by making state of art medical information available to more critical care professionals? One that is consistent with ethical guidelines concerning gifts to healthcare practitioners? Look no further, the Society of Critical Care Medicine has a practical way to demonstrate that your company cares about the patients it serves." If one did not know that the Web site belonged to a professional society, it could easily be mistaken for a commercial education enterprise.

The president of the society in 2002 refused to tell me whether consultants for industry are allowed to be officers of SCCM, how SCCM justified having its logos and name on virtually everything (including its publications) at its congress, and how, as a professional society, it justified crass commercial come-ons on its Web site. Her reply consisted mainly of a defense of SCCM's practices based on its compliance with the laws regulating nonprofit organizations.[47]

The Gastroenterologists

Another medical society that engages in hucksterism is the American Gastroenterological Association (AGA). Its annual Digestive Disease Week (DDW) meeting (held in Orlando, Florida, in 2003) offered for sale its shuttle buses, portfolio bags, and luggage tags, Internet stations, job-placement service, program books, badge lanyards, and hotel keycards, each for a hefty price. Their Web site breathlessly exclaimed, "Many companies sponsor the same DDW events and products from year to year, so act now! Take advantage of the world's largest GI meeting to advertise your company."[48]

But there are other examples of AGA's close industry ties. An "unrestricted" grant from Wyeth Pharmaceuticals permitted the AGA to produce a glossy-covered booklet called *Nocturnal GERD* (gastroesophageal reflux disease). The clock on the cover shows sheep calmly jumping a fence at 1:00 AM, and a fiery heartlike shape at 3:00 AM, signifying terrible middle-of-the-night heartburn. *Nocturnal GERD* is part of the Nighttime Heartburn Relief Effort, an official publication of the Digestive Health Initiative, the educational arm of the AGA. The brochure says, "The program was launched in response to a Gallup survey, commissioned by the AGA, that revealed 79 percent of heartburn sufferers experience symptoms at night."[49] (This will come as no surprise to any doctor.) In fact, Wyeth suggested the survey and paid for it.[50] Wyeth, incidentally, makes one of the prominent proton-pump inhibitors (Protonix), a mainstay of treatment for GERD and its complications. Other companies that make proton-pump inhibitors are Janssen, AstraZeneca, and TAP Pharmaceuticals. The AGA has a policy that prohibits corporate sponsors from having any involvement in development of the medical content of their products. Nonetheless, the chair of the six-person Nighttime Heartburn Relief Effort that produced the pamphlet is a consultant for Wyeth as well as two other proton-pump inhibitor manufacturers, and is on the speaker's bureau for four. Except for one, the remaining authors of *Nocturnal GERD* are either consultants, on the speaker's bureau, or have research grants from three of the four companies that make the drugs.[51] Given that *Nocturnal GERD* is an official publication, one can't help wondering why the AGA selected participants so closely connected to the manufacturers of proton-pump inhibitors.

The Endocrinologists

The Endocrine Society came under criticism for conflict of interest after it published its first clinical practice guideline, one that offered advice about testing and treating older men for testosterone deficiency. The diagnosis of testosterone deficiency is based in part on vague symptoms such as tiredness and reduced interest in sex, and also on measurements of testosterone hormone levels in the blood. Unfortunately, testosterone measurements in many laboratories are unreliable, and they vary considerably from hour to hour and day to day. Given the uncertainty in diagnosis when it is based on patients' symptoms and testosterone measurements, a serious quandary exists about treatment. Although certain preparations that contain testosterone can effectively raise the blood levels of the hormone, it's hard to know who should be treated. If medications for the conditions were without side effects, and if drug costs were negligible, the treatment decision would be an easy one, but it is not. Testosterone treatment accelerates the growth of prostate cancer, a condition that is common in the very same population of men in whom testosterone deficiency is most common.

The conflict of interest? Dr. Jerome Groopman, a physician and science writer, spelled it out in a 2002 article.[52] Groopman contrasted a 2001 report by a group of nonconflicted experts at the NIH with a 2001 report by the Endocrine Society. In short, the NIH group cited the difficulties in measuring testosterone, the lack of a well-proven way to make the diagnosis, and urged great caution in treating men suspected of having the condition until more research was available on testosterone blood levels and the effects of testosterone treatment.[53] By contrast, the Endocrine Society panel concluded that testosterone should be measured when hormone deficiency is suspected (they suggested all men over age 50), and that a course of testosterone treatment might be warranted even if testosterone levels were not low when a man's symptoms suggested hormone deficiency. Unfortunately, many members of the Endocrine Society panel had financial ties with Solvay, the company that markets AndroGel, a new (and already widely used) testosterone preparation that raises the level of testosterone in the blood when it is rubbed on the skin. In addition, Solvay supported the panel's work financially. Dr. Groopman also reported that Solvay had nominated members of the Endocrine Society's panel and some of the nominees were allowed to become panel members.[54] Clearly, many members of the Endocrine Society panel had a conflict of interest, but is their report biased? Dr. Groopman implied that it is.

But, the financial conflict of interest has a dimension not reported by Dr. Groopman: loosening the diagnostic criteria for testosterone deficiency and recommending more avid screening and follow-up for the disorder creates a new, large market of patients for endocrinologists. Given that the only large population who seek care from these subspecialists are patients with diabetes, the large number of elderly men who might be tested or treated could be a boon to the practice of endocrinology, a new market for urologists who do prostate biopsies to monitor for cancer, and a windfall to the companies that market testosterone blood tests and testosterone treatments.

In fairness, the panel recommendations were the first clinical practice guideline that the Endocrine Society had produced, and the society probably did not appreciate how skeptical many would view the recommendations of a panel that was funded by Solvay and that contained many members with financial arrangements with the company.

The Nephrologists

Nephrologists, or medical kidney specialists, have had complex relationships with industry ever since the costs of patients on dialysis or treated by kidney transplantation were first covered by Medicare 30 years ago. Conflict-of-interest issues surfaced decades ago when many nephrologists profiteered from the generous federal reimbursements by overcharging the government, selling their patients to commercial dialysis units, and running huge operations with shoestring budgets. In 1999, Dr. William Bennett, then president of the American Society of Nephrology (ASN), established a committee to define the key ethical issues in education, research, and clinical practice raised by the interaction of the profession and industry; conflict of interest was a central aspect to be assessed. The committee identified major conflicts of interest involving education, research, and patient care. Issues were raised about compensation of directors of dialysis units, the quality of care given to dialysis patients, the structure of research projects, financial incentives that tempt clinical investigators to pressure patients to participate in research, and influence by industry on educational efforts. The committee proposed that the council of the society obtain systematic data about the extent of the ethical problems and assess whether the con-

clusions of its preliminary report would be borne out by a more comprehensive study. Late in 2003, Dr. Bennett provided a follow-up. He said, "The
ASN decided not to pursue this matter further. I was outvoted 5 to 2. The
ASN and academic 'researchers' are far too tight with industry for me. I was
frustrated and took a great deal of flack from industry and colleagues for
even suggesting the issue."[55]

The Psychiatrists

Psychiatrists are latecomers to the drug-company money trough but they are
making up for lost time. Scattered through the book are examples of psychiatrists' strong industry ties. Until 1987, when Prozac was introduced, the
drug industry had little interest in collaborating with psychiatrists; the practice of psychiatry was dominated by psychotherapy—talking and analyzing—
not pharmacotherapy. The transformation of psychiatry since the
introduction of a new class of drugs, selective serotonin reuptake inhibitors
(SSRIs), that benefit many patients with anxiety, depression, and schizo-
phrenia, has been profound. (The SSRIs include widely prescribed drugs
such as Paxil, Lexapro, Zoloft, Celexa, and Effexor.) In combination with
the introduction of these drugs and restrictions by insurers of treatment
sessions for psychiatric illnesses, many psychiatrists have left talking sessions behind and become psychopharmacologists, experts in the use of the
new psychotropic drugs.

The pharmaceutical industry has fostered this transformation by engaging key academic psychiatrists and community opinion leaders as consultants, sponsoring clinical practice guideline committees,[56] and paying for
all kinds of educational venues for psychiatrists. In some academic psychiatry departments, virtually all of the educational meetings and meals are
paid for by one company or another. Dr. Marshall Folstein, former chair of
the Department of Psychiatry at Tufts University School of Medicine, told
me that drug testing has become widespread in medical centers and was
"destroying academic psychiatry departments."[57] In one of the most striking examples of individual psychiatrists' involvement with industry, Dr.
Folstein described an experience with one psychiatrist who offered to join
his department at no cost to the department if Dr. Folstein would put no

constraints on his personal financial involvements with industry. Folstein refused. He indicated that some psychiatrists were supplementing their salaries by $300,000 to $400,000 per year through their industry connections. Dr. Carol Nadelson, the former editor of the American Psychiatric Press, Inc. (APPI) and former president of the American Psychiatric Association (APA), said that, as with many other medical professional societies, the annual meeting of the APA is heavily subsidized by industry, as is the APPI.[58] She noted that many of the drug-company-sponsored symposia at the annual meeting of the APA are better attended than the scientific presentations. She indicated that she is deeply worried not only about the influence of industry in psychiatry, but by the evolving focus on money making in the APA.

One of the latest flaps in psychiatry circles that has spilled into the public press deals with the safety of the SSRIs. Occasional suicides and violent behavior in children have led to calls by some to follow the lead of the British equivalent of our FDA in banning all SSRIs for children except Prozac, and early in February 2004 the FDA was scheduled to hold hearings on the issue. Days before the hearing, a group of researchers from the American College of Neuropsychopharmacology, headed by two prominent academic psychiatrists, released a preliminary analysis of their Task Force on SSRIs and Suicidal Behavior in Youth. It concluded that antidepressants did not increase the suicide risk in children, and that the benefits of SSRIs outweighed their risks.[59] Their report was immediately criticized because nine of the ten panel members allegedly had "extensive ties to the pharmaceutical industry."[60] Some critics labeled their report "junk science"; others were less restrained.[61] At the hearing, FDA regulators testified that their analysis did suggest that in clinical trials the risk of suicide in children was increased over those taking placebos with some of the SSRIs.[62] So far, the FDA has decided only to require a warning about possible suicide tendencies in descriptions of these drugs.

The picture that emerges is a changed psychiatry profession: changed in part because of changes in the way psychiatric care is financed, and in part by the extraordinary influence of the pharmaceutical industry. The lives of many people have been improved vastly by these powerful, but sometimes dangerous, new drugs. But, as seen in the example of the Task Force, many are concerned that financial conflicts of interest may have a pernicious influence on the pronouncements of even high-placed academics, and that biases based on financial connections to industry can lead to devastating family tragedies.

The AMA

The grandfather of professional organizations, the 157-year-old American Medical Association, is "dedicated to be an essential part of the professional life of every physician" and to be "an essential force for progress in improving the nation's health." It has tried to set high standards of ethical conduct while attending to its members' interests, but the organization has not always been successful at doing both. During the twentieth century, the AMA was a force for good in advancing medical education, public health, and high quality of medical care. But the organization, like many others, has struggled to define its mission. Should it act as a guild, which primarily services its members' well-being (especially financial well-being), or should it aspire to higher ideals, which in turn might narrow these financial prospects? On the one hand, if an organization such as the AMA behaves as a guild, it loses respect as a professional organization. On the other, holding to the highest moral and ethical virtues and values may threaten its members' income and they may object and resign. In fact, membership in the AMA has fallen dramatically over the years. Though at one time approximately 70 percent of American physicians were members, now less than 40 percent are full dues-paying members.[63]

Though in the last half of the twentieth century the AMA has continued to advocate for better medical education, high standards of medical care, and improvements to public health, in one instance after another, it has seemed more intent on preserving political power and its members' income. Starting in the 1920s and continuing through the 1990s, the AMA opposed universal health coverage run or regulated by the federal government. It railed against "political medicine" and "socialized medicine" and claimed that the quality of care would fall, that governmental medicine would interpolate a politician between doctor and patient, and that doctors would become slaves of government. All efforts were made to preserve the status quo: namely, the ability of the doctor to set his own charges without governmental interference.[64] In the mid-1960s the AMA opposed Medicare, not appreciating at the time that the program later would reap great benefits to practicing doctors because of its generous fee-for-service structure. In the late 1980s as a move toward universal coverage strengthened, the AMA lobbied against it, and in the 1990s, the AMA helped defeat the Clinton health plan, complaining that it entailed too much government regulation. They were not alone; yet in each of these instances, the AMA was seen by many as self-serving.

An overt financial conflict of interest aroused the public's attention in the late 1990s when officers of the AMA made their deal with the Sunbeam Corporation to endorse nine household products in exchange for a royalty on each item sold. An immediate public outcry forced them to spend millions of dollars to extract the organization from the deal.[65] Still they did not learn. In 2001 the AMA launched a $645,000 educational campaign to convince physicians not to accept gifts from pharmaceutical companies. Unfortunately, the campaign was funded by grants from an "industry roundtable" consisting of Eli Lilly, Bayer Corp., GlaxoSmithKline, AstraZeneca International, Merck & Co., Pfizer, Inc. and Wyeth-Ayerst. The irony of accepting drug money to pay for a campaign against drug money seems to have been overlooked by AMA leaders. Support by the pharmaceutical industry for this kind of effort was widely criticized.[66] It is interesting to speculate on the motives of companies that seem to be spending money on programs that seem to act against their own best interests. Maybe they really want to "purify" the profession. Or one could be cynical and suppose that they are merely trying to sanitize their efforts in the eyes of the public.

What's Going On?

We know that the professional societies are heavily subsidized by industry, and that such subsidies reduce dues for members and allow the societies to carry out some of their educational and research missions. Yet we know little about the downside of these connections, namely what kind of influence these subsidies have on the policies and educational and clinical products of these professional societies. We also know virtually nothing about the possible financial conflicts of interest of officers of professional organizations. From the many complex arrangements, it is apparent that physicians and medical professional organizations with close financial ties to industry are intricately involved in developing clinical practice guidelines and a variety of new industry-sponsored pamphlets, books, Web sites, registries, and quality initiatives.

Why such heavy involvement? The most generous interpretation is that the involved physicians are "true believers," that they simply believe strongly that cholesterol-lowering drugs and the new anticlotting drugs should be used far more widely, that doctors aren't keeping up with the latest medical literature, and anything they can do to help educate them should be done, even if it requires getting funding from pharmaceutical companies that, in turn, will undoubtedly benefit from the wider drug use.

Or maybe disagreements between one group of experts and another, in the case of the use of the clot busters, is just a scientific kerfuffle; just a dispute over how many angels could fit on the head of a pin, and that each side is entitled to its opinion. From Wennberg's studies at Dartmouth, we know that the widest variations in how patients are treated are precisely in those areas in which the data can be interpreted in various ways. This, again, is a generous, neutral, possible interpretation.

But the money that changes hands between the companies on the one hand and individuals and professional organizations on the other suggests a darker, more serious, plausible interpretation. As the press has begun to write about financial conflicts in medicine and as the government has begun to promulgate rules about gifts, elegant dinners, and trips to fancy resorts, pharmaceutical companies have quietly switched their marketing strategies. They now try to influence the recommendations of practice guidelines developed by professional organizations with physicians financially connected to them who serve on clinical practice guideline committees and by supporting the organizations in other ways. They apparently have seduced high-placed physicians with financial rewards to collaborate with them to develop front organizations that produce Web sites, books, and registries, and to support lay advocacy groups that promote their products. Willingly or unwittingly, it appears that many physicians and some professional medical societies have become marketing agents for drug companies. In some sense, the drug "reps" of the past have been supplanted by academic physicians and "key opinion leaders" in the practicing community.

Harlan Krumholz, a cardiologist and researcher at Yale University, asked rhetorically: "What is the appropriate level of interactions? Should academics, who are widely perceived as objective, credible, trustworthy sources of information be enriched to a substantial extent through marketing efforts with pharmaceutical companies?"[67]

Doctors' associations have multiple roles. They advocate for good medical practice, promote their members' welfare, organize meetings of scientists and practitioners, support research, develop clinical practice guidelines, and lobby government to advance their agendas. Over time, medical professional organizations have come to depend increasingly on funds from industry to support their growing operations and mammoth meetings. In making these connections, some have compromised their role of serving the best interests of the public.

7

CAN YOU TRUST YOUR DOCTOR?

The intricate web of entanglements be-
tween doctors, medical organizations, and industry clearly affects the information that doctors rely on as they see their patients. But of course, the
encounters between doctors and patients are personal, involving a trust
unique to these relationships. This trust is based on the fundamental (and
centuries-old) assumption that the doctor places the welfare of his patients
at the very top of his priorities.

The task of putting the patient first has become far more challenging in
the modern era than it was 2,400 years ago when Hippocrates penned his
famous oath. In fact, the task has become more challenging than it was 47
years ago when I recited the oath, and especially more difficult since I
stopped practicing medicine in 1991 to take the reins of the *New England
Journal of Medicine.* The cost of becoming a doctor is considerably greater
now, yet many doctors' incomes have flattened out and some have even
fallen. Expectations of great financial success still exist, however, especially
in specialties in which procedures are a dominant part of the practice. There
is little doubt that the many ways that physicians are paid for their labors
can affect the choices they make in the day-to-day practice of medicine.

How Is Your Doctor Paid?

It goes without saying that a practicing physician's livelihood is integrally
linked to the care of patients. The physician receives compensation for providing a much-needed service, and for many years in the twentieth century,

patients paid their doctor bills out of their pockets, often in cash. Altruism often governed what form and how much payment doctors requested. This payment system was short lived as technology advanced, as treatments improved, as hospitals increasingly became the sites of care, and as new expensive medicines were developed. At the same time a system of medical insurance, funded largely by patients' employers, replaced out-of-pocket payments. Under this system, physicians no longer received compensation directly from patients, but billed insurers for the services, including office and hospital visits, and office tests they did themselves. Medical insurance allowed people to receive more and better care, but it also separated the payer from the recipient of health care and placed the physician smack in the middle.

The fee-for-service system was virtually the only payment system until the late 1970s. Until then, the insurance companies, and the government (through Medicare and Medicaid), paid for most of the services that doctors billed, and for a time, though some doctors "worked the system" and billed more than they should have, there was little clamor over the cost of care. In this fee-for-service (FFS) system, whatever the patient needed, the patient got. For a time, physicians' and patients' incentives were well aligned: the cost of care seemed reasonable, though steadily rising, and both patient and doctor were mutual beneficiaries of this approach to the organization and funding of the health-care system.

Needless to say, this mutually beneficial arrangement didn't last long because the fee-for-service system promoted an excessive use of services. Clinical decisions are not always black or white, and doctors often have considerable discretion in deciding whether to order a test or treatment in a given clinical situation. Well, they did order more tests and treatments; some were probably unnecessary and some of these were ordered to inflate the doctor's earnings. As a result, the cost of medical care began to rise rapidly and reached levels that most economists, not to mention employers, considered unsustainable. Much maligned today, managed care evolved as a way not only to control costs but also to manage the ever-increasing complexity of care. Managed care already had a long but sleepy tradition in the country (especially in California at Kaiser Permanente) when, in 1973, Congress gave the new mode of patient care a boost by legislation that fostered its growth, and in the mid-1980s managed care began a huge expansion.[1] The fundamental idea was simply that an insurance company would try to manage the care of the patients they insured in a more systematic way than under the uncontrolled and the apparently uncontrollable fee-for-service system. The idea was that the companies would pay only for services that were genuinely necessary and withhold payment when they were not.

In managed care, doctors are paid according to two main financial arrangements. The first is a full-time salary arrangement in which they are paid regardless of number of services they provide or the number of patients they care for. The second method is "capitation." Capitation was a new payment system based on care for a specific population of patients, not a specific patient. In capitation (or a capitated system), groups of physicians contract with a managed-care organization to take care of all the medical needs of a cohort of patients in exchange for a specified amount of money per member per month. Older managed-care organizations such as Kaiser in California and (the former) Harvard Community Health Plan in Boston traditionally paid their physicians a salary and often supplemented it with bonuses tied to productivity, as measured by the number of patients seen and the cost savings from efficient care. Care was generally managed by HMOs, and many variations of these HMOs came into existence. In some, physicians are employed and controlled directly by the HMO, in others, the HMO contracts for the care of their members with physician groups or with individual physicians in solo practice.

Over the years HMOs have used a variety of approaches to hold down the use and costs of services. They initially employed primary-care physicians as "gatekeepers" who were expected to restrict unnecessary and expensive tests and treatments. They urged primary-care physicians to learn enough gynecology, dermatology, and orthopaedics to avoid sending patients for consultations to specialists who were still generally paid on a fee-for-service basis. They hired cadres of physicians and nurses to review doctors' decisions before they were carried out (so-called utilization review). They created extensive profiles of the testing and treatment practices of physicians, and used these records to reward doctors financially when they saved money for the insurers and to punish them when they spent too much.

HMOs created monetary incentives for patients as well. If Medicare patients joined a Medicare HMO (that was less expensive than traditional Medicare), they would get a drug benefit that was unavailable under regular Medicare. In many HMOs, to reduce the use of doctors' services, patients were required to pay out of pocket a small copayment for every office visit.

For several years these strategies had a dramatic effect. The cost of medical care, which had been rising at a rate of 8 to 10 percent per year in the early 1990s, leveled off in the late 1990s at 2 to 3 percent.[2] And though criticism of and dissatisfaction with managed care grew, those who paid for health care (the employers and government) breathed a sigh of relief. But experts in health economics were not fooled. They predicted that the lull in inflation was only temporary and that given the rising costs of labor, technology, drugs, and the aging of the population, inflation would return. And by the end of the 1990s, it did.

Why is all of this organizational detail and cost information relevant to each individual patient's interaction with his doctor? The answer is simple. Every method of physician payment creates a financial conflict of interest for the doctor. In a fee-for-service system the doctor may be inclined to do more than is necessary for his patients if his income depends on how many visits he recommends and the number of tests he personally performs. In a capitated system, if the money the doctor spends on his patients' care threatens to reduce his earnings, he may be inclined to provide too few services for his cohort of patients. And physicians who are fully salaried may try to avoid seeing patients if their income is independent of the number of patients assigned to them. In short, there is no incentive-free system; money talks for physicians as it does for all of us. Thus, given one incentive or another, some safeguards are necessary in each system to prevent abuses stemming from the lure of financial gain.

The critical question is whether financial incentives distort physicians' decisions and injure patients. Certainly, doctors who deliberately decide to cheat the system can find ways to do so. An additional, important question is whether financial incentives warp the judgment of honest and well-intentioned doctors who may be subconsciously influenced in situations where the best clinical course of action for a particular patient is not clear. There is little doubt that such subconscious influences do exist and thus the judgment of even the most ethical physicians can be influenced by financial incentives. At the same time, any system must be careful not to impinge seriously on physicians' income: doctors must be paid well to insure that smart people are willing to go through the grueling schooling and training required to become a doctor in the first place.

The Fee-for-Service System

Cost and the quality of care are important issues, not just for the health-care system as a whole, but also for each patient who visits his doctor. In the fee-for-service mode, some doctors performed lucrative procedures on patients who didn't really need them (or in whom the indications for the procedures were fuzzy). Some performed unnecessary surgery. Some sold drugs and alternative medicine potions directly to patients. Some brought patients back for office visits more often than medically necessary. Some worked the system to get the highest possible return from drugs that they bought at wholesale and sold at retail.

Cardiac procedures were easily abused. Some doctors performed electrocardiograms and billed for them at every office visit even when the test was unnecessary. (One cardiologist estimated that a busy practitioner could perform as many as 70 to 80 in his office in a busy week.) And because the clinical indications for other cardiac tests, such as echocardiograms, stress tests, and heart catheterizations were not well specified and often changing, it was easy to justify doing more tests than necessary. These tests were also the ones with a large cash yield when applied to large numbers of patients. Whereas a doctor might get paid $16 to $18 in the 1980s and 1990s for performing an electrocardiogram in his office, he would receive an additional $25 to $30 for a cardiac stress test, and another $140 to $180 for an echocardiogram. In addition to the charge for the office visit, the extra tests could easily net an additional $200, and if the doctor carried out a heart catheterization, the fee would be an additional $450 to $500.[3] Many patients received all the tests, and went away feeling that they had been well treated, not realizing the waste of time and money involved.

Excessive testing hit the headlines in 2002, when the FBI raided the offices of Chae Hyun Moon, director of Cardiology, and Fidel Realyvasquez, Jr., chairman of Cardiac Surgery at the for-profit Redding Medical Center in Redding, California. Moon and Realyvasquez were suspected of performing unnecessary procedures, (including open-heart surgery!) and thus overcharging Medicare. Their colleagues claimed that 25 to 50 percent of the procedures they performed were unnecessary, and an independent assessment showed that the Redding Medical Center led the rest of California in the number of bypass surgeries performed per 1,000 Medicare enrollees.[4] Neither the FBI nor the state have filed charges against the physicians, and their attorneys contend that the investigation is unjustified.

Not surprisingly, the greatest ambiguity in the use of tests arises when the medical facts about the tradeoff between the risks and benefits of testing are still incomplete. A case in point is so-called whole-body scanning. In recent years some physicians, principally radiologists, have invested large sums of money to purchase private CT machines capable of scanning the entire body, and they have offered this service to the public, often through ads in the media. Health insurance doesn't cover the cost, but some people are willing to pay the $900 to $1,000 charge out of their pockets to have the scan.[5] Without a lot of medical knowledge, getting an image of all one's internal organs sounds like a good idea: if there is a hidden cancer or an unsuspected calcium deposit in some important artery, something might be done about it before it causes harm.

In fact, the harm of getting these scans is sometimes greater than the benefit. Although some potentially curable cancers and other disorders are occasionally found by such scanning, many findings are difficult to interpret, and as a consequence they may lead to attendant anxieties, unnecessary additional testing, and even unnecessary surgery. As with most tests, they have to be applied to the right populations to yield meaningful results, and we are not yet certain for which group the body scan would be most useful (if any). Despite these cautions, some physicians have promoted body scanning to the public.

The Tenacious Battle to Preserve Self-Referrals

The battle over self-referrals is an excellent example of the profession's struggle to deal with the conflict between physicians' income and optimal patient care. Patients who visit their doctors offices often need certain tests and treatments that cannot be administered on site, and their doctors have always sent them for these to local hospitals or to free-standing diagnostic and treatment centers in the community. During the 1980s, (in the final stages of the heyday of fee-for-service medicine) physicians could refer patients to testing and treatment facilities in which they were part owners. Thus, a patient who needed a specialized imaging study such as a CT scan, might be referred to an imaging center partly or fully owned by the doctor who sent the patient; and a patient who needed X-ray treatments for cancer might be sent to a facility owned by the referring oncologist. The free enterprise system worked rapidly and effectively. Commercial ambulatory surgical centers began to spring up everywhere. To increase facility use and compete with other similar facilities, these companies offered enterprising surgeons profits in the company or an ownership stake. One large hospital chain substantially increased the use of its operating rooms by sharing the profits with staff surgeons.[6] In another type of arrangement, ophthalmologists accepted financial inducements from manufacturers to use their intraocular lens implants in cataract surgery, in the form of quantity discounts, cash rebates, shares of stock, and gifts such as free vacations, the use of yachts, and expensive office equipment. Radiologists invested in free-standing radiologic imaging centers featuring CT scanners and MRIs, often in partnership with venture capitalists.[7]

The stage was set for overuse of the facilities. Eventually in 1989, the inspector general of the Department of Health and Human Services (DHHS) found that the Medicare patients of physicians who had ownership of the facilities received about 45 percent more laboratory services than patients whose doctors did not have such arrangements.[8] Self-referring primary-care physicians who sent patients for imaging studies in offices in which they had a part ownership ordered about four times more examinations for the same medical problems as compared to physicians who referred patients to independent radiologists. The self-referring physicians also billed more for similar imaging studies relative to the radiologists. This combination of more frequent testing and higher charges resulted in a 4.4 to 7.5 times higher average charge per episode of care.[9]

In another study, when the use of magnetic resonance imaging (MRI) and CT scans in three Florida cities (where 93 percent of the imaging facilities were privately owned) was compared with Baltimore (where almost none of the facilities were privately owned), the rates of use in Florida were 65 percent higher for MRIs and 28 percent higher for CT scans.[10] Leaders of the AMA contested the significance of these studies and the others described before, but Representative Pete Stark of California held hearings that culminated in a law aimed at ending self-referral. Representative Stark argued that, no matter how well intentioned, such arrangements involved a serious conflict of interest that threatened the doctor-patient relationship. He felt that self-referral puts patients in a position where they would be forced to question their doctor's advice and loyalty.[11]

During the 1980s, as self-referral spread, the American Medical Association declared that such arrangements were not unethical as long as the physician disclosed the relationship to his patients. The AMA argued that physicians should not be prohibited from investing in or participating in the ownership of facilities within health care. It believed that such a policy was restrictive and would impose unnecessary and unfair economic discrimination against its members. The AMA claimed that restricting self- referral would adversely affect the access to care, that it would inhibit innovation, and would harm efforts to improve the quality of care. There was little evidence for these concerns, but there was already considerable evidence that self-referral increased the cost of care.

In 1991 the AMA Council on Ethical and Judicial Affairs proposed a voluntary halt to self-referral, but six months later, by an overwhelming vote of the AMA's house of delegates, the rank-and-file members approved a resolution approving self-referral as long as the arrangements were disclosed. (They did so over the objections of their own Board of Trustees and their Council on Ethical and Judicial Affairs.) Eventually, Representative Stark prevailed: legislation was passed in the mid-1990s and was implemented over the next five or six years. The antikickback provisions barred any remuneration to induce patient referrals. The Stark bills covered many different services, including clinical laboratory testing, occupational therapy services, X-rays, and radiation therapy. Violators could be punished by ex-

clusion from reimbursement from Medicare and Medicaid, but also pros-
ecuted for a criminal offense.[12]

Managing Care and Managed Care

Slightly more than one-quarter of Americans are enrolled in HMOs. Much
of the public resentment against managed care relates to the perception
that it restricts care to enhance profits. In fact, many plans, particularly not-
for-profit, older plans, were created to provide health care for patients over
long periods in a more rational and less costly way. For most of these, cost
containment was not the primary purpose. An initial principle of these plans,
which unfortunately was hard to sustain, was to accumulate a cohesive group
of physicians who agreed with a single philosophy of care and would not
need excessive rules and controls to manage the care. Most patients enrolled in these plans were greatly satisfied with their care.[13]

Managed care has special advantages, and many practicing physicians
acknowledge that managed care in their hands has made them provide
better care than their previous "unmanaged" care because of the demands
that health plans make in the way preventive services and treatment of patients is monitored. Physicians should also welcome the fact that many of the
excesses of the fee-for-service system have been left behind, including indi-
vidualism and autonomy as a fundamental principle for the approach to everyday medical practice, uncritical differences in practice style, paternalism
as a mode of decision making, and self-centeredness instead of evidence as
a basis for medical decisions. The managed-care movement has also forced
us to realize substantial benefits of the changes in the way medical care is
delivered. We are now paying much more attention to the measurement of
the quality of care, to the long-term management of chronic diseases, to
the cohesion of care, prevention of unnecessary hospitalizations, to super-
fluous and unnecessary testing, to excessively expensive treatments, to the
satisfaction of patients, and to the costs and appropriateness of our routine
medical interventions. It is unlikely that we would have made as much
progress in many of these areas without the pressure from managed care.

Policy makers hoped that managed care would control the tests and treatments that doctors order and contain out-of-control increases in medical

costs. The challenge of financing health care centers in part on managing "risk," that is, coping with the cost of care and trying to keep it under certain limits. In fee-for-service plans the insurers bear the financial risk. Under capitation, physicians (or physicians' groups) bear the risk. Now, in yet another attempt to exert control over increases in the cost of care, the insurance industry is passing an increasing portion of the risk to patients in the form of copayments. What this means is that patients are increasingly bearing more of the financial burden of their care, over and above the costs that their insurance plan covers.

Managed care became particularly nettlesome to doctors and patients because of the controls it placed on both. Doctors resented the role of gatekeeper because it inserted them between the patient and his or her care. They bristled at the requirement to get permission to refer to specialists and to order certain tests, and although this requirement all but disappeared several years ago because of the anger about it, it is reappearing.[14] When monitoring of care was done after the fact, as it often is today, many doctors take umbrage at having their decisions second-guessed. Shifting some of the financial risk from managed-care companies (which are principally insurers) to the physicians who perform or order the care also can create bad will. As noted before, under capitation, physicians are paid a fixed monthly price to provide care for a panel of patients. If they spend less, they keep the remaining funds, but if they spend almost all of the allocation on their patients' care, little or nothing may be left for them. There are also other financial incentives that limit physicians' use of resources and threaten patient care. These include bonuses for keeping down costs and withholding part of a physician's income until the end of the year in case they overspend their allotment. Needless to say, all of these financial arrangements that put the physician's income at risk pit the doctor's responsibility to provide optimal care against his personal financial welfare.[15]

Most physicians do not like capitation and prefer to work in a fee-for-service system, even though most of them realize that the costs of such care are impossible to control. Nonetheless, capitation in some form or another is almost certainly here to stay. The issue is whether the conflicts of interest associated with capitation, and the finite resources we have to spend on health care, can be managed so that patients are protected against inappropriately restrictive care.

Financial Incentives to Restrict Care Do Work

Financial incentives to restrict care keep costs down and minimize overuse of services. Salaried physicians hospitalize their patients less frequently than physicians paid in a fee-for-service mode, and physicians who work in a capitated arrangement hospitalize patients even less.[16] Hospital lengths of stay in capitated models are remarkably short, and despite the short stays, there is little evidence that the quality of the care such patients receive is compromised (though patients and their families are often more inconvenienced).[17] Placing physicians at financial risk reduces testing and referrals to specialists. But reducing services requires making judgments that are difficult, often not clear-cut, and unpopular with patients. Given the ambiguity in medical information and medical decision making, denying care in some instances can be quite arbitrary.

In a study of more than 700 physicians selected randomly, almost one-third admitted that they sometimes had not offered patients useful services that were not covered by their health plan. Only 42 percent said that they never had withheld such options.[18] Too much testing or treating invites criticism. Vincent Kerr, the former director of Healthcare Management at the Ford Motor Company, told me in mid-2003 that a physician organization in the Detroit area threatened to expel several physicians from the group because they were "outliers" when it came to the costs of the care they provided.[19]

The problem is exacerbated in health-care plans owned and operated by physicians who treat patients and at the same time decide on whether to pay claims and receive year-end bonuses according to cost savings. Such incentives induce cost-consciousness and conflicts of interest that can lead physicians to alter their medical advice to patients. People generally understand that such restrictions are necessary, but when it comes to their own care, or the care of a family member, they often want more care, not less. (In fact, many are actually better off with less.)

Managed-care organizations want to keep their customers happy and convince them to remain as paying customers, but when profitability is an overriding motive, compromises are bound to happen. Unfortunately, when premiums rise, some patients may have to give up coverage or switch to less expensive plans even though it may require losing a long-standing relationship with their physician. In fact, patients are often unable to judge when their care is being short-changed. They often do not have sufficient information on which plans offer better services, and when they are acutely ill, their judgment may not be sound.

Supporters claim that the remedy to managed care's incentive-driven restriction of medical care and less candid advice about treatments not covered by the plans lies not only with the insurer's desire to keep their customers satisfied, but with the physician's professional ethical obligations to his patients. We know by now from a variety of other situations in which physicians have financial conflicts, however, that not all doctors can be counted on to uphold their ethical obligations.

Many physicians complain that under managed care, they have less time for patients, they are perceived by patients as adversaries because of their gatekeeping roles, and they have less ability to place their patient's interest first. More than half of physicians in one survey were negative toward managed care, about 30 percent were neutral, and only 5 percent were positive.[20] The respondents in this survey were mostly older physicians many of whom had experience with the system before managed care. Presumably, younger physicians who have known only managed care, and have adjusted to its administrative requirements and financial restrictions would be less negative.

The Ethical Dilemmas of Restricting Care

A critical negative consequence of managed care is the extraordinary pressure it exerts on the integrity of practicing doctors. As the rate of growth of patient-care funds available from the government, from employers, and from insurers slows, the temptation of physicians to protect their incomes has grown, and as more care is tightly managed, and as more physicians are expected to pay attention to the overall health and expenses of a panel of patients, the temptation to undertest and undertreat is substantial. In this setting, financial conflicts of interest exist that pit the ethical behavior of a physician toward his or her patients against the physician's personal finances. This conflict can threaten the physician's loyalty to the patient.[21]

Less than ten years ago physicians were expected by managed-care executives to withhold information about the benefits of health plans from patients (the so-called gag rule). When I was editor of the *New England Journal of Medicine*, I published one example that created quite a stir. Cambridge (Massachusetts) physicians Stephanie Woolhandler and David Himmelstein described one contract with U.S. Healthcare HMO that stated, "Physicians shall agree not to take any action or make any communication which undermines or could undermine the confidence of enrollees, potential enrollees, their employers, their unions, or the public in U.S. Healthcare or the quality of U.S. Healthcare coverage. . . . Physician shall keep the Proprietary Information [payment rates, utilization-review procedures, etc.] and this Agreement strictly confidential."[22] Even though most companies no longer require physicians to abide by such gag rules, insurance company managers may exert subtle pressure on doctors that deter them from telling their patients what a plan does and does not offer.

When physicians are under pressure to limit the cost of their patients' care, they can easily be torn in their loyalties to their patients and especially to their own families, because with one or two false moves they can be out of a job. These divided loyalties that threaten a physician's livelihood are wrenching. The incentive for doctors to preserve their jobs may be so strong that they may no longer be willing to act exclusively as the patient's advocate. They may even be unwilling to go to bat for the patient with the management of an HMO when they think that a given service is needed but is being restricted inappropriately. Anybody placed under such stress would be unable to tolerate it for long: this situation could produce an even greater threat, namely a loss of integrity. Some physicians might find themselves conforming to the restrictions and deceiving themselves into thinking that what they are doing is best for the patient when in fact they are providing suboptimal care. In short, they would be living a lie.

The physician under pressure who is medically responsible for the care of a panel of patients and at the same time is in financial jeopardy ("at risk") when he fails to minimize costs faces a special dilemma. Rather than adhere to the time-honored principle that at the bedside or in the office, each patient comes first, the physician is expected to adopt a "distributive" ethic, which upholds the principle of providing the greatest good for the greatest number of patients within an allotted budget.[23] The conflict between caring for one versus caring for a group creates an obvious conflict that can create difficult choices, and it is not clear that the individual patient always wins out. Many feel strongly that the focus must always remain on the individual patient, and that allocation decisions must not be made at the bedside.[24]

Under managed care (and in some fee-for-service arrangements as well), physicians face another ethical dilemma, namely what to do when the insurer sets certain rules that the physician believes are not in the patient's best interest. Examples of such imposed conflicts include changes in formularies and restrictions on certain therapies. The conflict arises because the physician can jeopardize his income, and even his job if he opts to use the treatment that is "outside" the plan's offerings. Unfortunately, requests to insurance-plan officials for exceptions to the rules often go unheeded.

Damaged Trust

Because the public perceived that managed care was all about restricting care, saving money, and making profits for the big insurance companies and their stockholders, people began to lose faith in the health plans and the doctors that practiced in them. It was not uncommon in the 1990s for doctors and patients alike to refer to managed care as "damaged care." (A movie of the same name hit the theaters in 2002.) Patient care may have been damaged somewhat during the growth of managed care, but the trust of patients in health care, and in doctors in particular, was damaged even more. A colleague, Dr. Wendy Levinson, described an experience that I heard from many others as patients became aware that doctors were being paid to restrict care.[25] She described one of her patients who developed arm pain after bicycling through rough terrain. Believing it was due to a nerve impingement in the neck, she recommended inexpensive nonsteroidal anti-inflammatory drugs and avoidance of certain kinds of physical activity. One week later, the patient returned in greater pain, involving both her neck and left arm. Because the patient's examination was again negative, Dr. Levinson and the patient agreed to pursue chiropractic treatment. The patient was not heard from for some time, but two months later, the patient returned with undiminished pain that was now keeping her up at night. This time, Dr. Levinson referred the woman to a neurosurgeon; eventually the patient underwent surgery and her pain was relieved. After some time, the patient returned to Dr. Levinson for a different problem, but shocked the doctor by asking, "Does my insurance company pay you not to refer? I've read in the newspaper about financial incentives for doctors to decrease the cost of care." Dr. Levinson was shaken: the cost of referring the patient to a specialist had not entered into her decision making.

Managed care was especially undermined by public disclosures of patients who claimed that their care was shortchanged because of attempts to cut costs. One such widely publicized case was that of Cynthia Herdrich, who came to her physician, Lori Pegram, for abdominal pain in March 1991 and was found to have an inflamed mass in her abdomen. Dr. Pegram ordered an ultrasound to confirm the diagnosis, but did not order the procedure at the local hospital. Instead, she decided that the patient could wait eight more days for the test to be performed at a facility 50 miles away that was staffed by her HMO.[26] Unfortunately before the test was done, Ms. Herdrich's appendix ruptured, and she was taken to surgery.[27] The patient recovered, sued her doctor for malpractice (and won the case), but also sued her HMO, CarleCare. The physicians who provided care to the HMO members not only owned the HMO, but also their professional medical-practice corporation and the management company that coordinated its activities, and the physicians received year-end bonuses based on the HMO's profits.[28] Ms. Herdrich argued in the suit that Dr. Pegram's financial and ownership ties with the HMO created a conflict of interest between personal profit and what was best for the patient. Ms. Herdrich's suit went all the way to the Supreme Court. The Court made this point:

> In this case, . . . one could argue that Pegram's decision to wait before getting an ultrasound for Herdrich, and her insistence that the ultrasound be done at a distant facility owned by Carle, reflected an interest in

limiting the HMO's expenses, which blinded her to the need for immediate diagnosis and treatment.[29]

Mrs. Herdrich lost the case because the Court did not believe that existing laws were sufficient to hold the HMO responsible for her outcome, but the publicity in her case and other similar instances of cost cutting by HMOs damaged the reputation of all of managed care.

In both of these examples and in many other public cases around the same time, patients lost trust in their doctors and in HMOs because of their perceptions that some doctors' actions in limiting testing or treatment were motivated by a financial incentive to limit care.

Trust is an important cornerstone in all kinds of human interactions, including familial, religious, social, political, and commercial. Medical trust is a centerpiece in patient-doctor relationships. Unlike many other forms of trust, medical trust stems from the intense vulnerability of people when they become ill. It is akin to trust in love or friendship, in that there is a strong emotional component, and the relationship is valued based on the understanding that the doctor will do the right thing for the patient. Mark Hall, professor of law at Wake Forest University, describes trust as "the core, defining characteristic of the doctor-patient relationship—the 'glue' that holds the relationship together and makes it possible. Trust is shown to be essential and unavoidable in medical relationships because patients need and want to trust, and without trust medical relationships never form or are entirely dysfunctional."[30] Hall points out that trust has a therapeutic benefit in and of itself and enhances the effects of treatment: although the therapeutic benefits of trust are not easily measured or quantified, many believe that they are real.

Trust declined in many professions during the twentieth century. In a random national telephone survey of more than 1,000 patients, 95 percent of the respondents said that they trusted their physicians, but 73 percent responded that it was a bad idea to give doctors a 10 percent bonus for cost control. Most said that they would choose a health plan without bonuses over one with a cost-control bonus. Moreover, 91 percent of respondents favored disclosure of financial information.[31] Even with such disclosure, however, the perception of conflict of interest might not be lessened. In fact, it might even be enhanced.

Profiting From Machines, Gadgets, and Implants

For 30 years the federal government has paid the bill for dialysis treatments under Medicare. At present, more than 200,000 patients with chronic kidney failure undergo dialysis in the United States. The cost of caring for these patients, including kidney transplantation, is now nearly $16 billion per year.[32] Early in the program the fees paid for dialysis were overly generous and many for-profit companies rushed into the business of providing regular treatments to patients with advanced kidney disease. Payments for dialysis include fees for physician supervision, for nursing and technical services, for drugs, for the numbers of patients served, and the kind of dialysis provided. In the early days of the Medicare program, some physicians took advantage of the generous payments and many rapidly became millionaires. Some left academic medical centers and started up their own independent for-profit dialysis units, and some academic physicians were reputed to have transferred their patients to existing for-profit centers for fees as high as $50,000 each. Currently, approximately 75 percent of patients receive their dialysis in private for-profit facilities.[33]

Over the years the Medicare program gradually reduced its payments (adjusted for inflation the decrease was approximately 64 percent over the past two decades) until at present many not-for-profit dialysis centers are having considerable difficulty surviving financially.[34] Nonetheless, for-profit dialysis centers still operate at a profit. Those who operate the investor-owned dialysis facilities argue that they are quicker to respond to newly emerging healthcare needs and they have lower costs than units in the not-for-profit sector. Still, many worry that lower costs in the for-profit facilities also means lower quality of care. The investor-owned dialysis units tend to employ fewer personnel per dialysis treatment, dialyze for shorter periods of time, and use less highly skilled personnel to staff their units. In terms of certain outcomes such as mortality rates and referral for transplantation, some find the for-profit units lacking, but others have found few differences.[35] The impact of dialysis unit ownership on patient well-being and patients' capacity to function from day to day has not been systematically assessed.

At the inception of this program, only a few people imagined how much the program would grow, how much it would cost, and how some physicians would take advantage of the generous payment system.

Devices such as implants, catheters, and stents (metallic devices that keep tube-shaped structures such as blood vessels and ureters open) have become essential therapeutic tools; without them we would be sicker, more disabled, and the quality of our lives would be lessened. But financial motives can also be the basis for their excessive or inappropriate use. Two of the most commonly used classes of devices used in day-to-day practice are those used by cardiologists and orthopaedic surgeons. Stephen Klaidman's recent book details the conflicts of interest faced by a group of inventive cardiologists who helped develop the modern tools of interventional cardiology, and there is no need to describe these conflicts in detail here. In short, Klaidman describes examples of cardiologists who use procedures inappropriately and excessively, resulting in unnecessarily high cost of care (not to mention the untoward side effects that patients suffer when an unnecessary procedure causes a complication). He gives examples of cardiologists who invent new devices and license them to established companies, some who start new companies and then sell them, and some that acquire large equity stakes in companies that make devices. Klaidman raises special concern about those cardiologists who have a direct financial stake in the products that they are developing and testing clinically.[36]

Klaidman and others have particular concerns about the crass commercialism of Transcatheter Cardiovascular Therapeutics (TCT), a private group that sponsors a yearly conference on various cardiovascular devices. Because the organizers of these meetings fund them privately, their meetings have none of the safeguards that characterize ordinary CME courses (such as a requirement to disclose financial ties and proscriptions against the discussion of unapproved uses of drugs and devices). As a consequence, speakers openly promote products. The conference attracts thousands of participants, and its principal organizer, Dr. Martin Leon, a New York cardiologist who has multiple financial ties with device companies,[37] holds forth and praises products himself. One cardiologist who attended a meeting described a kind of circus atmosphere, with three screens, two for the content of a talk and one for advertising relevant products. As venal as some of the medical societies meetings are, TCT's tilt to the device companies are described as much worse. There is little doubt that many interventional cardiologists, especially many of the participants in TCT, have substantial ties to device companies.

The device industry in orthopaedics is a multibillion-dollar operation that includes such company giants as Johnson and Johnson, Zimmer, and Smith and Nephew. Orthopaedists help these companies develop implants that make worn out, damaged, and diseased joints and bones work again. The orthopaedists also help make various kinds of equipment that help them perform their specialized surgical procedures. To develop the devices and equipment, orthopaedists often work with small companies that have expertise in the kinds of materials necessary for constructing new implants and devices, and many are rewarded with company stock or stock options. Once developed and approved, the orthopaedists are free not only to use them on their own patients, but also to recommend their use to other surgeons. Dr. James Herndon, 2003 president of the American Academy of Orthopaedic Surgeons (AAOS) that encompasses 18,000 surgeons, told me that these arrangements are a setup for abuse, in part because of substantial uncertainties in his field about which devices and implants are optimal to use.

There exist too few careful evidence-based studies in orthopaedics to make judgments about the optimal use of these devices. As a consequence, devices can readily be overused and inappropriately used. Dr. Herndon pointed out that long after new and improved implants have come available, some surgeons continue to use their own outdated implants, which generates substantial personal profits. And through consultations with companies, ownership of stock, and lectures that include products, Dr. Herndon explained, some orthopaedists can supplement their clinical incomes by as much as one to two million dollars per year.[38] The AAOS code of ethics requires its members to disclose to patients any financial arrangement with a durable medical goods provider, royalties from patents, and any "significant" gift from industry.[39] How often AAOS's members or other orthopaedists follow these guidelines is not known.

Disclosure of Financial Incentives in Direct Patient Care

At first glance, it would appear that, for patients, the solution to understanding and dealing with the incentives of physicians in a health plan is to receive full disclosure about how the plan's physicians are paid. In fact, such openness could also deter health plans from using incentives that would be difficult to justify in public. Unfortunately, because disclosure can have both positive and negative effects on a doctor-patient relationship, a great deal more work must be done to determine how best to heighten the positive effects and diminish the negative ones. On the positive side, disclosure can "inform enrollees' choice of plan, reinforce enrollees' capacity to understand and exercise other rights under managed care, and discourage use of compensation methods that might compromise patients' access to treatment."[40] In addition, it is quite clear that, given the option, patients do want to know about incentives. On the negative side, however, evidence suggests that patients are made uncomfortable when forced to think of the physician-patient relationship in financial terms. Further, the complexity of many plans' systems of reimbursement make them difficult to understand.[41] Most worrisome, of course, is that disclosure may undermine the perception of a physician's trustworthiness.[42]

Some government agencies have begun to force the issue. States began to force disclosure of physicians' financial incentives in 1995, with 28 states requiring disclosure by the end of 1998. In 1999, President Bill Clinton ordered all federal agencies to institute disclosure of physician incentives, though current federal laws require disclosure of incentives only if a patient asks.[43] Managed-care plans under Medicaid and Medicare cannot apply incentives designed to reduce or limit medically necessary services (however, such decisions are not always clear cut).

Incentives Based on Quality of Care

As part of movement away from financial incentives that limit expensive tests and procedures, several employers and health plans in Massachusetts, Ohio, and Kentucky are launching bonus programs based on the quality of care their physicians deliver.[44] They measure quality by checking doctors' patient records. For example, if a doctor does a good job controlling blood pressure, cholesterol, and blood sugar in his diabetic patients and becomes a member of the American Diabetes Association's provider recognition program, he will receive an additional $100 per patient each year. In Massachusetts, Blue Cross and Blue Shield began to award 8,000 doctors cash bonuses for above-average jobs of caring for patients while also providing cost-efficient care. Once the program is fully implemented, a group could earn up to 15 percent in addition to total regular fees in a given year, which it could divide among its doctors. Doctors will also receive payments for establishing electronic medical records, systems for tracking the care of chronically ill patients, and developing patient-education programs. Several California plans are starting similar initiatives. In that state, where much care is capitated, physicians will be able to qualify for a $2 per member per month bonus if they meet six patient satisfaction and medical care standards.[45]

However, there is disagreement over what measures should be used to determine quality, how much incentive is meaningful, and whether bonuses will be based on giving money to some doctors and taking it away from others.[46] Some have proposed that physicians' performance be judged against national clinical practice guidelines, but the costs of adhering to guidelines that regularly identify underutilization of expensive drugs may call an early halt to such programs. We can also expect that doctors will work to achieve whatever quality measures are devised, and will provide improved care to the extent that these measures accurately reflect real health-care quality. The idea of giving extra payments for better quality of care is an interesting one. On one hand, each physician should already be providing the best care for each of his patients, and thus no incentive for the best care should be necessary. And yet it is clear that optimal care is not always given. Further, such financial incentives may have a beneficial effect by calling attention to specific kinds of high-quality care.

Incentive payments based on quality or consumer satisfaction probably will represent less than 10 percent of doctors' total income.[47] This fraction may be too small to have an impact on the average physician. Thus, although there is a popular movement toward giving bonuses based on the quality of care, they will have limited impact on financial conflicts of interest if they are dwarfed by the power of other incentives. It is much too early in the "pay-for-quality" agenda to guess whether the concept is sustainable.

Advice for Physicians

Mark Hall has suggested common-sense principles for physicians, namely to avoid entering into incentive arrangements that they are embarrassed to describe accurately to their patients, and to appraise honestly whether financial incentives are excessive. He suggests that physicians should be wary of incentive arrangements that are not in common use elsewhere in the market, even though common use doesn't guarantee that such arrangements are acceptable. Hall warns that doctors "should not steer their patients into different insurance plans according to arrangements that will produce the most physician revenue: sick patients into fee-for-service, healthy ones into capitated plans." He points out, this "may not harm the patient," but is "inappropriate manipulation of varying payment structures for the physician's benefit."[48]

Advice for Patients

Unfortunately, our medical-care system is imperfect, and many patients are limited in the kinds of health plans they can afford. If cost containment continues, as it undoubtedly will, and if physicians continue to bear some of the financial risk for the care they give, as many almost certainly will, some strain in the trust between doctor and patient, though regrettable, is probably inevitable. Patients must appreciate that because of the inherent characteristics of the system, their doctors are pushed harder than ever to see more patients in a shorter time and encouraged to conserve resources as the cost of medical care continues to increase. Patients will have to take more responsibility for understanding what their plans offer and what they exclude. When possible, they should choose a plan after understanding the principal financial implications of joining. Regrettably, this is often a tall order given the complexity of these arrangements.

Nonetheless, patients are not powerless just because they are forced into one plan or another. They can ask whether their physicians receive bonuses or other payments for constraining cost, how difficult it is for their doctor to refer them to a specialist, and whether their doctor needs special permission to do so. They can ask whether their doctor's financial performance is monitored, and if so, what use is made of the information. They can try to learn whether major financial decisions about care are the responsibility of business managers or physicians: in the final analysis, even physicians burdened by incentives are better judges than managers of how to avoid compromising patient care. Finally, patients could try to assess whether physicians in the plan advocate for their patients when coverage decisions are questionable or when desirable tests, medications, or other treatments are not covered by their health plan.

How much can a patient be expected to do, anyway? *Caveat emptor* may be an appropriate slogan for selling used cars or life insurance, but it is not a worthy dictum for health care. In the final analysis, it is not a patient's responsibility to protect himself against the medical profession, it is the profession's responsibility to protect the patient. Doctors have a responsibility to help patients understand their recommendations. Especially when they are withholding certain tests or treatments or recommending inexpensive ones over the latest highly publicized ones, physicians have an obligation to explain the rationale of their actions to their patients. Furthermore, they have an obligation to go to bat for the patient if some procedure or treatment is not offered by the patient's plan, but is one that would contribute importantly to the patient's health and welfare. These are some of the ways that physicians can maintain the bond of trust with their patients in this complex and imperfect system.

There is no physician-payment system that is free of financial incentives; fee-for-service promotes overtesting and overtreating, and capitation does the opposite. Both systems produce ethical dilemmas for physicians and can create distrust of doctors, but doctors and patients distrust capitation more. Disclosure of incentives in patient care, though no panacea, can make financial arrangements more transparent. Ultimately, the physician must bear the responsibility to act in his patient's best interests.

8

CAN WE TRUST OUR RESEARCHERS?

THE BENEFITS OF MEDICAL RESEARCH, IN-
cluding those in collaboration with industry, have been truly astonishing.
In the 50 years since I started medical school, advances in diagnosis and
treatment have revolutionized the practice of medicine. When I started to
practice, diagnostic methods were primitive. To visualize the brain, doctors
had to inject air or another substance into the spinal canal, a painful procedure. Now it is done from outside the body with CT and MRI scans. Diseases that could not be diagnosed accurately in their early stages, such as
multiple sclerosis, are routinely identified (and treated) now. Diseases of
the pancreas and biliary tree could be diagnosed only by exploratory surgery; now they are identified with scans and long tubes that have miniature
lights and cameras at their ends. The cause of heart attacks could only be
inferred; now the artery blockage can be seen and corrected, and many
heart attacks are now preventable. New treatments have revolutionized the
management of certain diseases. Transplants of kidneys, livers, and hearts
have become routine, and successful. Some malignant diseases such as
Hodgkin's disease, testicular cancer, leukemia, and tumors of pregnancy
are curable. AIDS, at first a nearly uniformly fatal disease, has been converted into a chronic disease. Medical devices save lives and improve life's
quality. Implantable devices shock irregular hearts back to regularity. Arthritic
hips and knees are routinely replaced. To a substantial extent, our free-
enterprise system and the promise of profits has encouraged physicians,
entrepreneurs, and commercial enterprise to invest their time and capital
in the search of new modes of diagnosis and therapy. It would be counterproductive to inhibit this inventive spirit.

Medical research has become an enormous enterprise in the United States. The federal government spent approximately 20 billion dollars in 2001 on it, and private industry spent even more: in the range of $30 billion.[1] The pharmaceutical industry's share of investment in biomedical research and development, now approximately 60 percent, has doubled since 1980. Today, approximately one-quarter of academic biomedical researchers receive industry funding.[2] In the sluggish economy at the beginning of the twenty-first century, medical research was one of the few areas of growth. Stockholders of pharmaceutical companies have much to gain as well as much to lose from the successes and failures of new discoveries, from newly approved drugs, and from expiration of patents on existing drugs. Well-paid executives of these companies have their careers at stake. Physicians who carry out the clinical trials for the pharmaceutical industry stand to gain much, both financially and in terms of their reputations when their studies are successful and are published in major journals. Governmental agencies vie for their share of the federal medical-research pie and for the publicity that successful clinical trials generate. Finally, and certainly not least important, ordinary people may benefit (and often do benefit) from the products of research.

Competing financial interests are not just hypothetical concerns. They can hurt research subjects, embarrass researchers, and severely damage an institution's reputation. Even one or two widely publicized research fiascos involving financial conflicts can spoil the trust of the public in our entire research enterprise. It goes without saying that without the trust of the public, clinical research could not proceed.

Falling Behind the Japanese

Concerned about the nation's economy and alert to what seemed at the time to be an unstoppable wave of Japanese entrepreneurial success, Congress passed the Patent and Trademarks Amendments Act (the "Bayh-Dole Act") in 1980 to stimulate the transfer of inventions and discoveries into commercial applications.[3] The act provided that universities would automatically receive patents for inventions and discoveries based on research sponsored by the federal government. Prior to the act few researchers or universities filed for patents. The idea behind a more aggressive policy was not new: many recalled the successful collaboration of academia and industry during the Second World War in the development of the atomic bomb and in the production of penicillin for battlefield infections. Like the 1980s Japan's economic miracle, the underlying secret seemed to be to tightly integrate business efforts and governmental policy. It marked the beginning of a national belief, which crystallized decades later, that for-profit enterprises and markets could solve many of society's problems.

The Bayh-Dole Act encouraged university researchers to innovate, prepare patent applications, and support the development and evaluation of resulting products. The university generally retains the patent to a given innovation, licenses it for a fee to one or more commercial enterprises, and industry then attempts to use the invention to develop profitable products. In turn, for their involvement in generating the invention or discovery and helping to develop a marketable product, profits that derive from licensing the patent are required by law to be shared with the inventor.[4] This association between academia and industry provided a new avenue to profits for researchers and institutions alike. The academic scientist, lured by the promise of royalties, became an entrepreneur, and universities became more like big businesses than centers for learning how to cure the sick.

In the past, in days that now seem hopelessly naïve, clinician researchers were motivated at the outset by a curiosity and zeal that was unscathed by a dream of fortune. At that time, even when an investigator developed a new invention or idea, the seeking of a substantial source of capital to finance development was particularly arduous. Today, on the other hand, investigators may find themselves pitching potentially marketable discoveries to eager venture capitalists even before they complete their preliminary studies. The process can be a heady experience.

Of course, these academic-industry collaborations have a downside. As early as 1980, some observers were already raising concerns[5] that investigators would pursue only those areas of research that promised riches, that students might be neglected, and that because of the expense of using patented materials, some investigators might not be able to carry out research that would otherwise benefit patients.[6] (Similar concerns were later raised about the patenting of genes.) Concerns about conflicts in the role of leaders of medical centers (deans of medical schools and presidents of medical centers) have also been raised. Because they have a vested interest in the success of their staff and faculty in converting their scientific discoveries into profitable inventions and products, these leaders might be too lax in the way they rein in the research projects of their faculty, particularly patient-centered research.[7] In itself, the opportunity for faculty members and institutions to profit substantially from discoveries and inventions creates an ideal environment for financial conflicts of interest.

The fast-paced, market-driven collaboration in clinical research raises concerns about the safety of patients who participate in clinical trials. To some extent, inventors of devices (and to a lesser extent, discoverers of new drugs) are the ideal individuals to test the new devices in clinical trials because they have the most concentrated expertise. Yet, the potential financial gain of positive results of the research can create the potential for patient risk, bias in the design of the research, and bias in the interpretation of the results. For these reasons, most new guidelines for the conduct of clinical research contain proscriptions against researchers carrying out human studies on their own inventions.[8]

A Watershed Event

The death of 17-year-old Jesse Gelsinger in 1999 during a research experiment at the University of Pennsylvania brought the intersection of clinical research and financial conflict of interest into sharp public focus. One reporter called it a defining moment for gene therapy. In fact, it was also a defining moment for honest and open discussion of the conflicts inherent in clinical research. Mr. Gelsinger had a rare genetic disorder of metabolism in which his cells were deficient in an enzyme (a protein) called ornithine transcarbamylase. In its most severe form, the condition causes early death in infants. Because his enzyme deficiency was mild, he had done well on a low-protein diet and medications, but he volunteered for the experiment even though he knew that he would not benefit personally from it. The idea of the experiment was to administer normal genes containing the enzyme, and to do so, the genes were imbedded in a common-cold virus. The experiment was designed to determine whether the treatment was safe;

a secondary but scientifically important question was whether the new genes would begin to make the enzyme. Although some experimental primates had developed serious side effects from the "treatment," including organ failures and even deaths, these adverse events were not reported to Jesse Gelsinger, Jesse's father, or the F.D.A. One human who had received the virus had few side effects, but Jesse developed lung, liver, and kidney failure, and died four days after receiving his first dose of the genetically engineered viruses.[9]

At first, Jesse's parents defended Dr. James Wilson, the principal investigator, but their sentiments soured when they heard that the gene therapy had been publicly described as a "treatment" even though researchers had not yet garnered any proof of its efficacy. They were even more troubled when they learned that both Dr. Wilson and the University of Pennsylvania had a financial stake in the outcome of the therapy.[10] Both Dr. Wilson and the university held stock in Genovo, Inc., a biotechnology company that Dr. Wilson had founded in 1992 and had provided 20 percent of Dr. Wilson's annual research budget for the gene-therapy experiments.[11] In return for its funding contribution, Genovo would receive exclusive rights to develop any of Dr. Wilson's research results into commercial products. Both Dr. Wilson and the university stood to gain financially from subsequent approval of the treatment, since both owned equity in Genovo.[12]

Jesse's parents wondered whether financial considerations might have spurred the investigator to test the therapy prematurely, or at least to test it in a boy only mildly affected by the disease rather than in a more severely affected infant. Dr. Wilson, the university, and Genovo all denied that the obvious financial conflict of interest contributed to Mr. Gelsinger's death, yet the university's Conflict of Interest Standing Committee (CISC) had predicted just such a quandary four years earlier when it reviewed the university's ties to Genovo. In an eerie prediction, a CISC panel had asked, "Since Dr. Wilson's research efforts will be directed towards the solution of a problem in which he has a financial interest in the outcome, how can Dr. Wilson assure the university that he will not be conflicted when making decisions that could have an impact on . . . his intellectual property?" Notably, the committee did not seek to have the financial arrangement terminated.[13]

The Gelsinger incident launched a nationwide investigation by the National Institutes of Health into gene-therapy trials as well as other clinical-research efforts, uncovering hundreds of unreported violations in research protocols and a number of injuries to patients, including several deaths. The case also led to calls for better methods to deal with financial conflicts of interest involving researchers and their institutions. Eventually the university settled with the Gelsinger family; the university survived its fiscal loss and the vast negative publicity, but there was an interesting postscript. One year after Jesse's death, both Wilson and the university made a profit on the commercial arrangement when a larger company bought Genovo. Reportedly, the university netted $1.4 million, and Wilson retained stock options worth $13.4 million.[14]

After Jesse died, Dr. Wilson adamantly denied being influenced by financial considerations, but in an interview he said, "To suggest that I acted or was influenced by money is really offensive to me. I don't think about how my doing this work is going to make me rich. It's about leadership and notoriety and accomplishment. Publishing in first-rate journals. That's what turns us on. You've got to be on the cutting edge and take risks if you're going to stay on top."[15] He said it wasn't about the money. Does he protest too much?

The arrangement that lead to Jesse's death was not only completely legal, it had been sanctioned for 20 years by none other than the federal government, with the expectation that patenting and licensing of inventions would benefit patients and spur business activity.

More Black Eyes

Around the time of Jesse Gelsinger's death, other instances involving financial conflicts of interest in clinical research emerged. In 1999, Roger Darke died during a gene-therapy experiment at St. Elizabeth's Medical Center in Brighton, Massachusetts. Mr. Darke had agreed to be part of a research project in which a gene for blood-vessel growth would be implanted into his damaged heart. If successful, it might suggest ways to improve the function of damaged hearts. In information that emerged following a lawsuit, it turned out that, unbeknownst to Mr. Darke, another subject in the same study had died a few months earlier. Darke's widow angrily said that her husband never would have participated in the experiment if he had been made aware of this or if he had been aware that the principal investigator, the late Dr. Jeffrey Isner (a Tufts University medical researcher) had a financial stake in the study's outcome.[16] The FDA later found that Dr. Isner delayed in reporting the first death to the appropriate oversight board, and continued to enroll patients in the study, thereby endangering patients' safety. Dr. Isner had collaborated with the hospital and several private companies to form a company called Vascular Genetics to support his genetics research. According to documents filed in the lawsuit, Dr. Isner owned 20 percent of Vascular Genetics, the hospital owned 20 percent, and the rest was held by several companies.[17] Mrs. Darke said, "As lay people we assume doctors in research are doing this for the betterment of mankind. But in this case there were billions of dollars that could have been made. That was something I felt we had a right to know."[18] When Dr. Isner was asked whether his financial connections might have influenced him, he made a comment quite different from Dr. Wilson's. He said, "I'm not going to be a wimp and roll over because someone is projecting a concern. I understand what the arguments are, but quite frankly, I don't agree with them."[19] Although the FDA shut down the studies at St. Elizabeth's Hospital for a short time,[20] it later allowed the experiments to resume when the institution reassured them that steps were being taken to minimize risks to patients.

Another widely publicized controversial research effort involved the Fred Hutchinson Cancer Research Center in Seattle. The "Hutch" had a respected reputation for innovation and success based on its pioneering work in the field of bone-marrow transplantation for leukemia. In one clinical trial intended to prevent a feared complication of such transplants, the donor marrow was infused along with manmade antibodies.[21] The sequence of those antibodies was owned by Genetic Systems Company, a Seattle biotech company that stood to profit from commercialization of the new technology, which it was testing on patients at the Hutch, and some of the doctors at the Hutch (and the Hutch itself) had financial ties to Genetic Systems. The three main investigators in the leukemia trial were Dr. E. Donnall Thomas, the clinical director of the Hutch (winner of the 1990 Nobel Prize in medicine); Dr. John A. Hansen, and Dr. Paul J. Martin. It was later revealed that Dr. Thomas held 100,000 shares of the company's stock, received a $3,000 annual stipend, and was a member of the company's advisory board. Dr. Hansen held 250,000 shares, had an $18,000 consulting contract, and a job as the company's medical director. Dr. Martin held 10,000 shares and had a three-year consulting contract. According to the reports, neither these financial interests nor the financial stake of the institution in the company were mentioned to the institutional review board at the time the proposal, known as Protocol 126, was filed.[22] The investigators claimed that they had never been told about the existence of the Hutch's conflict-of-interest policy, and said that their work did not directly bear on the business workings of Genetic Systems.

In a trial on behalf of five patients who died during this clinical trial, the jury found the Hutch not negligent in four of the deaths. After the trial, however, the jury's foreman said that the most compelling argument made by the patients' families was that the doctors owned shares of stock in a company whose antibodies they were testing. But the trial judge did not consider these financial arrangements sufficient to justify a charge of fraud and had thrown out the charge.[23] The Hutch has denied all allegations of wrongdoing, but by the time of the trial the Hutch's Board of Directors had already revised their conflict-of-interest policy to provide for greater transparency. In addition, the changes "expressly prohibit a Center scientist from being involved in a human subject trial if he/she has certain financial interests in a for-profit sponsor that could be impacted by the outcome of the trial. These prohibited financial interests include shares of stock in any amount, royalty rights on patents or other intellectual property, and payments which exceed $10,000 per year from a single entity."[24]

Conflict-of-interest policies vary widely among major biomedical research institutions across the country.[25] Dr. David Korn, the former dean of Stanford University Medical School, noted that "A remarkable feature of U.S. science policy during the past 50 years has been the relatively light hand of federal oversight of the scientific process and the deference shown to scientific and academic self-governance, which, in turn, rests on sustained trust in the integrity of faculty and scientists."[26] As seen in the above examples, trust sometimes is not sufficient.

Community-Based Clinical Research

Clinical trials can be long and expensive, and physicians often have difficulty finding enough patients who match the study criteria. Pharmaceutical companies, dissatisfied with the pace of clinical trials, began encouraging
entrepreneurial practicing physicians to help populate the rosters of their
clinical trials. The number of private-practice physicians engaged in drug
studies nearly tripled from about 4,000 in 1990 to more than 11,000 in
1997.[27] Between 1991 and 1998, the percentage of industry money for clinical trials at academic medical centers declined from 80 to 40.[28] Clinical
researchers are no longer found exclusively within the ivy-lined gates of top
universities—these days they also operate out of group practices, HMOs,
and even offices in strip malls. Tempted by faxes and letters with "blaring
come-ons" such as "Improve Your Cash Flow," some doctors have taken the
bait, which can exceed several thousand dollars per patient enrolled. The
process becomes even more attractive when multipatient bonuses are offered, such as a recent offer by Merck, which promised doctors an extra
$2,000 if their "quota" of 14 patients was enrolled by a certain date. With
incentives that approach $1 million a year for the most enterprising physi-
cians, some doctors at the fringe have turned their practices into virtual
contract-research organizations.[29] There has been little public debate over
clinical research because contactual agreements typically forbid doctors to
disclose their activities, and their methods are generally framed as proprietary trade secrets.

Given the lack of training in research among practicing physicians, concern has been raised about the accuracy and validity of some clinical trials
conducted in the communities. During the 1990s, nearly three-quarters of
physicians who conducted clinical trials had been involved in three or fewer
previous trials, a figure unlikely to give them mastery over the process. For
the most part, the only people practicing physicians have to guide them are
representatives of the companies sponsoring the research. Moreover, many
such clinicians are generalists, and not necessarily well trained to assess
complex responses to drugs. One odd result of the recruiting frenzy is that
specialists have also found themselves conducting activities ill suited to their
training, and even dangerous to the patient. In one instance, an asthma

specialist dispensed experimental medications for psychiatric disorders. And psychiatrist Dr. Claudia Baldassano, who conducted a trial on hormone replacement, was asked to conduct Pap smears. "I said I hadn't done a Pap smear since medical school," she said. On another occasion, she was asked to treat patients with diabetes.[30]

Kurt Eichenwald and Gina Kolata, *New York Times* reporters who have uncovered many excesses of clinical research, reported in 1999 that Dr. Peter Arcan recommended that one of his patients, Thomas Parham, a retired metalworker in La Habra, California, enroll in a trial for a drug designed to shrink enlarged prostates, despite Mr. Parham's objection that his prostate was healthy. Dr. Arcan suggested that Mr. Parham begin the trial anyway, stating that the new drug may have preventative properties (in fact, it might have had). What Dr. Arcan did not tell his patient was that SmithKline Beecham (now GlaxoSmithKline), had offered him $1,610 for each patient he enrolled. Nor did Dr. Arcan tell him that his heart condition disqualified him for the study, even after he complained of fatigue two weeks after beginning the trial. Dr. Arcan had managed to enroll him in the trial anyway after obtaining an exemption from SmithKline; he told the drug company's representative that Mr. Parham's heart condition was mild, and neglected to tell them that he had in fact been hospitalized for it the previous year.[31] Several weeks later, Mr. Parham left the study and later required a pacemaker. Whether Mr. Parham's participation in the study negatively affected his heart condition is not known. What is clear is that it was inappropriate for Dr. Arcan to enroll him in the trial. We have no idea how often patients are squeezed into a study for which they do not qualify, or how often financial incentives motivate inappropriate enrollment. In addition, although investigators are expected to report adverse events that occur during the course of a trial to the FDA, such reporting is uneven, sometimes grossly flawed, and occasionally overtly deceptive. Some drug companies are known to be parties to this deception.

The incentive structure of clinical trials often pits individual physicians against one another in an "arms race" to secure a roster of enrollees. One special perquisite offered occasionally to doctors who recruit the most patients is the right to claim authorship of a study, even where many physicians participated, and the true writer is a ghost author. Dr. Jay Grossman, a respiratory specialist in private practice in Tucson, Arizona, said he had been credited with authorship on more than one study for which he was the top patient recruiter, although he rarely did any of the actual writing, stating, "That's common."[32]

Because of their academic standing and reputations, physicians at medical centers have at least a chance of warding off inappropriate conditions (such as flawed study design, lack of control of study data, inappropriate selection of placebos, changes in submitted manuscripts, and control over whether a negative study is published) imposed on them by industry sponsors. Physicians in the community are less likely to be able to stand up to such demands. A major detractor of research in the community, Dr. Sidney Wolfe, views these commercial drug trial networks as "handmaidens of the pharmaceutical companies, concerned with the approval and marketing of drugs, rather than with true science."[33]

Enrolling patients in a clinical trial (whether in an academic center or in the community) can be a subtle form of coercion. A patient's trust in a doctor and his desire not to anger or offend the physician can make it nearly impossible to resist an invitation to participate in a study. Patients fear that by refusing to participate, they will anger their doctor and possibly receive suboptimal care. Even the highly sophisticated health economist, Princeton professor Uwe Reinhardt, said that he agreed to participate in a clinical trial conducted by his doctor because he did not want to annoy him. Reinhardt wrote "You want to keep his favor. If you say no, you'll worry that he may not like you."[34] As happens to many other patients who become participants in clinical trials, Professor Reinhardt had not been told that his doctor had been paid to recruit him. Although patients are required to sign consent forms, the forms do not account for any interpersonal pressures involved in the consent process.

What Are the Regulators Doing?

The OHRP (Office for Human Research Protections of the United States Department of Health and Human Services), the FDA (Food and Drug Administration), and IRBs are responsible for protecting human subjects in clinical trials. Any given trial may be subject to the regulations and review of all three. These oversight bodies are responsible not only for conflict of interest but for reporting requirements, data review, adherence to inclusion criteria, and other compliance issues. The blossoming of clinical research since the OHRP was founded and a lack of commensurate blossoming in resources has left the agency seriously overworked and unable to carry out its policing function effectively. By 2002, the agency was operating on a budget of only $7.3 million, but was responsible for overseeing tens of thousands of studies at more than 4,000 federally funded institutions.[35]

Even if the OHRP were adequately funded, its power would be limited. Its regulations require that institutions maintain a conflict of interest policy, designate someone to monitor disclosure statements, and establish enforcement mechanisms and sanctions where appropriate. But the agency has been hampered in developing stringent conflict-of-interest policies because of opposition from the pharmaceutical industry and some academic leaders who worry about hindering academic innovation, (and possibly losing income from their faculty's patents?). In fact, OHRP has not issued regulations, only "guidance." In their guidance, they actually admit, "Despite these . . . regulations, there is currently no uniform, comprehensive approach to consideration of potential financial conflict of interest in human research." Clearly, the OHRP guidance falls far short of being a clear mandate for individual conduct. It asks only that "[c]linical investigators *should* consider the *potential* effect that having a financial relationship of any kind with a commercial sponsor of a study might have on his or her conduct of a clinical trial or interactions with research subjects" (emphases added).[36]

Many commentators find that the existing regulatory structure, for its confusion, overlap, internal contradictions, lack of specificity, oversight, and consequences, is wholly "unreliable as a mechanism to police against conflicts of interest."[37] The present system relies too heavily on good will and self-regulation among both institutions and individuals. Where oversight is delegated, it is often given to the already overwhelmed and underfunded IRBs, which may not have the resources to monitor financial arrangements as well as clinical parameters.

In one study of 250 federally funded institutions, 6 percent had no internal conflict-of-interest policy and only 1 percent required disclosure to either IRBs or experimental subjects.[38] Dr. Bernard Lo at the University of

California at San Francisco studied the internal conflict-of-interest regulations of ten major universities, and discovered that while all had a disclosure policy regarding conflict of interest, the requirements for which
researchers had to disclose, what they had to disclose, and to whom they
had to disclose varied dramatically. Only four institutions required all members of the research staff to disclose. Only one of the ten institutions prohibited investigators and research staff from holding stock, stock options,
or decision-making positions in a company that might be affected by the
work. Dr. Lo found that although institutions are required to establish sanctions, they might be as minimal as asking the physician to reflect on whether
his conflict could give rise to bias. He also cited several instances in which
the policies that governed a small number of industry-sponsored clinical
trials were substantially stronger than conflict-of-interest policies in some
medical schools.[39] Unfortunately, most industry-supported clinical trials do
not meet such a high standard.

Many suggestions have been made to improve the oversight of clinical
research, and some deal specifically with financial conflicts. One strategy
to manage the conflicts would be to transfer a researcher's equity in a particular company to a blind trust for the duration of his involvement in a
study.[40] The Association of American Medical Colleges has also issued useful recommendations for dealing with financial conflicts of interest in clinical research.[41] The guidelines are high minded but also voluntary, so that
academic institutions need not implement them, and all policing (if any) is
done at the local level. A helpful recommendation from a physician group
in Boston proposed that researchers from academic institutions should not
be allowed to retain their full-time faculty status and at the same time take
a leadership role in a new for-profit company outside the institution.[42] The
proposal proscribes physician-inventors from evaluating their own drug or
device discoveries.

Harvard Medical School's official policies, approved in June 2004, are
perhaps the most stringent of any in the country.[43] Harvard researchers are
not permitted to have a financial interest in a company and conduct clinical research on a technology owned or obligated to that company. Harvard's
full-time researchers are also not allowed to hold executive positions (including scientific director and medical director) in any for-profit biomedi-

cal company. The rules do not, however, bar faculty members from consulting for industry, from serving on industry advisory boards, from becoming paid speakers for industry, or from receiving royalties for their inventions.[44]

Effects on the Research Enterprise

Pharmaceutical and biotechnology companies invent new testing equipment, biologics, and drugs. They produce many of the drugs that keep us healthy, free of pain, and cure our serious ills. They tell us on TV to ask our doctors if drug X or Y is right for us. At the same time, they are in business to make a profit, and they offer generous financial incentives to investigators and institutions to perform their clinical studies. This collaboration produces wonderful drugs that allow us to live longer and better. Unfortunately, it also produces many adverse consequences: enrollment of patients unqualified as subjects, falsified research results, and overt harm to patients by overzealous investigators.[45] One pair said, "The enormous legal and financial power of the pharmaceutical industry puts clinical investigators in a very difficult position if there is a major controversy about the outcome of a particular study."[46] The consequences of this power imbalance and the financial incentives given to investigators on the kind of research done and on the outcome of the work could be enormous.

Financial incentives can and do influence how study questions are framed and the very design of experiments.[47] Studies show that industry preferentially supports trial designs that favor positive results.[48] Some investigators for industry intentionally compare their new drugs to placebo controls when the appropriate control is the best available treatment. Comparisons can also be staged between the new drug and a drug that is not a perfect fit with the symptoms in question. Doses of comparison drugs can be rigged to favor a new drug, and duration of treatment can be carefully selected to favor a new drug. Some studies narrow the range of observations of side effects. Often the principal investigator simply has little role in a study's design, and just receives prepackaged instructions from the company. Outside investigators summoned to review the protocol may be brought in "pro forma."[49] The very nature of the contractual relationship between physician investigators and drug companies can be problematic. As a condition of the contract, researchers may be forced to sign away their right to monitor and control data, to analyze the data, and even to notify institutional overseers if something goes wrong.

In 2001, major medical journals (including the *Annals of Internal Medicine, JAMA, New England Journal of Medicine,* and the British journal, *Lancet*) provided some help to authors who carry out studies for pharmaceutical companies. They declared that they would not "review or publish articles based on studies that are conducted under conditions that allow the sponsor to have sole control of the data or to withhold publication."[50] They do not specify, however, that the authors should have control over the design of studies, which, as described above, can be biased in favor of a favorable outcome for a company; all they require is that "Authors should describe the role of the study's sponsor(s), if any, in study design."[51]

Frequently, when the investigator does retain control over the initial study design, his proposal must be approved first by the company's marketing division. For example, a company may insist that the drug be tested in a healthier or younger group of subjects, or on disease sufferers whose ailments are in a certain phase, compared to those who will eventually receive the drug.[52] Independent physician investigators who challenge the design can be fired from their assignment or not hired back. In doing so, they may acquire a negative reputation among other drug companies as well, for not being "cooperative" enough.

Delays in publishing, choices in research topics, and withholding of information are a few of the negative consequences of industry-supported research. Others include withholding information to delay dissemination of an undesirable result,[53] and keeping research results secret even beyond the time needed to file patents, presumably to protect proprietary information.[54] Finally, there is considerable evidence that some industry-supported research is biased.[55] Sheldon Krimsky's recent book ably describes the potential negative consequences of financial conflicts to the research and academic enterprises.[56]

Advice for Patients

Unfortunately, patients will have to ask hard questions of doctors who want them to participate in clinical-research projects. Is the doctor's payment for enrolling patients based on a quota system? Have there been any adverse reactions in previous subjects, including animals? How will my response be monitored? What reactions and side effects might occur? Patients must be assertive in reporting changes to the investigator and any other physician they may be seeing. If a patient enrolled in a clinical trial is unable to get solid, believable answers from the doctor carrying out the trial, they should seek the opinion of another physician who has no involvement in the research project.

Although patients would do well to heed this advice, they should not have to be so alert to their own welfare in clinical-research efforts. Clinical investigators must insure that their experiments minimize any risk to their research subjects.

Fostering the medical research enterprise is one of the highest priorities of the profession. Recent high-profile examples of financial conflict of interest in some major research centers threaten to undermine the public's trust of all medical research. Clinical studies are no longer only the province of academic institutions, and widespread research efforts in the community are inadequately regulated. People who participate in clinical studies must be fully informed of all potential risks.

9

HOW DID IT HAPPEN?

How did we get here? How did money come to exert such a remarkable influence over the medical profession? Is Luke Fildes' famous painting of a pensive doctor sitting patiently at the bedside of a sick child in bygone days only a fleeting fantasy?[1]

Half a century ago, medical centers were few in number, as were full-time researchers and teachers. Researchers, without the financial incentives available today, worked hard in their laboratories because of their passion for discovery, and professors (at least the ones I encountered) passed on their clinical skills because of their love of teaching. But it was also a much less sophisticated time. Few truly valuable drugs were available, diagnostic tests were primitive, and doctors had plenty of time to comfort, to teach, and to explain. Medicine was the most respected profession in the country. The federal government had virtually no involvement in health care. Except for the few full-time physicians at the very top, most were underpaid, and they stuck to the academic life for its substantial personal, nonfinancial rewards. The best researchers rigorously eschewed any relations with industry. The small cadre of full-timers were the icons of their time: crowds of physicians and trainees showed up at the yearly medical scientific gathering in Atlantic City for their lectures, for which they were paid with admiration and respect, bordering sometimes on reverence.

In this long-past era doctors in practice seemed also more innocent, more giving, and more altruistic. Most were self-employed, and thoroughly ensconced in a full-time local community practice. Only a few specialties existed at the time, and specialty medicine was not a dominant mode of care.

Private practitioners had virtually full control over their work: they were paid whatever they asked for in fees directly out-of-pocket by their patients. Many doctors worked long hours and realized great satisfaction for the small improvements in health they were able to achieve with their limited tools. There was a tradition to give substantial time to the care of the indigent, and in exchange many doctors accepted just tokens for their services. Medicine has always been recognized as part business, part profession, and although the credo "the patient comes first" was not always honored, it was an important ideal to which the profession aspired. Louis Brandeis captured the credo when he described a profession as follows, "it is an occupation which is pursued largely for others and not merely for one's self; . . . it is an occupation in which the amount of financial return is not the accepted measure of success."

An Ancient Problem

The clash between the doctor as wage earner and the doctor as healer, with its attendant compromises, was recognized in the times of the ancient Greeks and Romans. In 1847 it was the subject of commentary in the *Boston Medical and Surgical Journal*, the *New England Journal of Medicine's* predecessor:

> That it is a profession in which an opportunity is presented for exercising the natural philanthropic yearnings of the human heart, chastened and heightened by a profound sense of Christian duty towards suffering humanity, must be admitted; but to pretend that a man takes upon himself the ceaseless labors of a medical practitioner for no other earthly motive than to prescribe drugs, as the greatest of earthly blessings, is positively ridiculous, besides being untrue. Such a physician would fain make it appear that his charities were in proportion to the weight and measure of his doses. The fact is simply this, that the practitioner of medicine has a stomach to be filled, a body to be clothed, and in most cases a family to maintain—and a variety of relations which he bears to the whole community, renders it positively necessary that he should conform to the usages of civilized society. To do so there must be an adequate income from some source to meet the expense of being part and parcel of the general population.[2]

Suspicion of doctors' pecuniary motives continued through the twentieth century. In *Long Day's Journey Into Night*, written in 1941, Eugene O'Neill shows his contempt for them. Edmund, one of his characters, has an ill-defined illness, and his mother contemptuously says, "Doctor Hardy! I wouldn't believe a thing he said, if he swore on a stack of Bibles! I know what doctors are. They're all alike. Anything, they don't care what, to keep you coming to them." (Act 1)[3]

Later, when Edmund is found to be suffering from consumption (tuberculosis) and has to go to a sanitarium, his miserly father says, "Who said that you had to go to this Hilltown place? . . . I don't give a damn what it costs. All I care about is to have you get well. Don't call me a stinking miser, just because I don't want doctors to think I'm a millionaire they can swindle." (Act 4)[4]

Soon thereafter the same issue caught the attention of *Fortune* magazine. In an article titled, "The M.D.'s are Off Their Pedestal," in 1954, it said:

> It [rascality in the medical profession] has various symptoms, but underlying them, say the men who have nothing to hide, is a persistent money mania. A physician, for instance, may engage in clandestine fee splitting. He may prescribe long series of expensive but needless shots. He may take on too many patients and compensate for his overloading by keeping sketchy records. He may take advantage of Blue Cross, Blue Shield, and other insurance plans by shipping patients off for costly and unnecessary hospital treatment—a procedure that crowds hospitals and jeopardizes the plans themselves. He may, if he is a city practitioner without membership on a hospital staff, keep on treating patients he lacks training to treat and delay referring them to a hospital or a clinic. And if he does surgery, he may maintain what can be the worst abomination of all, his own profit-making hospital where there are no colleagues to check on his performance.[5]

And another half-century later we continued to worry about the same issues. As historian David Rothman opined, "There is considerable interest in reinvigorating medical professionalism. This interest reflects a profound unease with the seeming primacy of economic factors among those currently affecting medical practice in the United States. There is general agreement that patients' interests must take precedence over physicians' financial self-interest and that professionalism also entails service to vulnerable populations and civic engagement. But as commentators focus on managed care and other issues of the moment, many considerations are entirely overlooked. These omissions may well subvert the effort to make professionalism relevant to contemporary medicine."[6]

Many in the profession are seriously concerned that some physicians are willingly violating their integrity in personal profit-making ventures at the expense of patients' welfare. These excesses are not new, but they are far more widespread today than in the past, and their consequences are more profound. To find an explanation for the evolution of the profession over the past 50 years is no easy task. It is not enough to focus on the enormous increase in the amount of money that changes hands within and outside of the practice of medicine or just the scope of financial conflicts of interest, but as well on the societal and medical environment in which these changes took place.

Many complex interwoven factors and events shaped today's health-care system. Not surprisingly, money has constantly influenced the directions our system has taken.

Molding the Modern Practitioner

The practice of medicine in the 20 years following midcentury changed drastically. The government subsidized hospital construction and, based on the perception that there was a doctor shortage, began to pay medical schools to increase the size of their classes. Increasingly, students in medical schools turned away from general medical fields and sought training as specialists. National Institutes of Health programs facilitated this switch by funding training grants to medical centers, under the assumption that more specialists and subspecialists were needed. Within a decade or so, local hospitals were able to attract gastroenterologists, nephrologists, and surgical subspecialists: ophthalmologists, neurosurgeons, and cardiac surgeons. Many of the changes we see today occurred as a consequence of government intervention, modifications in the mode of practice, and a new influence of market factors.

Perhaps the most powerful influence, however, was the introduction of health insurance and the use of "fringe benefits" as a tool for employee retention and recruitment. During the era of price controls in the Nixon administration, employers were unable to preserve their work force and avoid strikes by offering workers higher wages (raises were frozen), but they were able to add fringe benefits, and health insurance was a powerful component of this new fringe-benefit package. Blue Cross/Blue Shield was one of the earliest insurers, but some early health maintenance organizations were also in operation, mainly in the West. The enactment of Medicare, however, in the mid-1960s, signaled a profound change in payment for medical care. For the first time, the federal government offered to pay for the medical expenses of an entire segment of the population, those over age 65. Those covered could now choose their own doctors and go for their medical care to any hospital, and doctors could now collect a fee from Medicare (or a patient's private insurer) for every service. Even the poor had access to insurance through Medicaid for some, if not all services. Doctors were reimbursed not only for office visits, but also for laboratory tests and special office procedures such as EKGs and chest X-rays. Practitioners' incomes benefited from these governmental programs. Until 1965 the average physician in practice earned about twice as much as the income of the average gainfully employed worker, but by the 1990s (despite managed care's restrictions) the figure had climbed to a multiple greater than five. There is little doubt that the enactment of Medicare and Medicaid improved the health of an enormous number of citizens and saved many from losing their life savings. At the same time, however, the combination of fee-for-service medicine and a rapidly expanding number of physicians who not only charged for office visits and in-office tests but also an evolving array of diagnostic tests such as CT scans, cardiac echograms, and colonoscopy rapidly helped to drive up the cost of medical care.

Suspicion was widespread that too many tests were being ordered and that physicians were encouraging their patients to return for more office visits than were medically necessary. It became a bit of a joke at the New England Medical Center, where I have worked for more than 40 years, that the house staff could tell when a patient had been referred into the center's cardiac service by a particular physician, all of whose patients sent in for cardiac catheterization had already had an EKG, a cardiac stress test, and a cardiac echo. They knew that not all of these tests were necessary in every patient. Other instances in which physician excess was documented were the practices of physicians who referred patients to testing and treatment facilities that the physicians partially or completely owned, such as rehabilitation facilities and X-ray laboratories. The assurance of payment for providing medical services either by private insurance or Medicare had a profound, unanticipated effect: doctors and facilities that could provide such services were more or less assured of payment.

Despite Medicare's strengths: wide coverage, improved care for the elderly, and low administrative costs, assurance of a payment for every service had another unforeseen and unintended consequence. It drove much of the charitable ethos out of medicine. Medical practice in the community and in academic medical centers always carried with it an implicit obligation for physicians to devote some of their time to the care of the underprivileged. In fact, at midcentury, academic medical centers were among the most respected of the philanthropic institutions. Many practitioners still give their time to the underserved without compensation, but discussions of charitable obligations often take a back seat now not only in institution board rooms but in many medical school conference rooms, where rising costs and survival now dominate the agendas.

During the 1970s the cost of care became a lightning rod for reformers armed with evidence that medical practice was not the sophisticated, scientific discipline generally accepted by the public, but one that relied more on physicians' judgment and experience than on well-documented facts. There is considerable disagreement whether the cost of medical care at that time (or even in our own time) is too much for our economy to bear, yet what mattered a great deal at the time was the *perception* that costs were excessive and uncontrollable. Thus, runaway costs and seemingly irrational clinical practices were powerful stimuli to restrict coverage for services, to develop benchmarks for payment, and to introduce administrative reviews of medical decisions. By the 1980s the judgment of the practitioner was no longer the last word in practice. The increasing costs also encouraged an approach to practice that already had achieved a foothold, namely health maintenance organizations (HMOs). As it turned out, money once again became a dominant factor in the new scheme.

HMOs began 50 years ago. When they came into prominence in the 1970s and 1980s, many had been conceived in an idealistic model to provide a more efficient alternative to the fee-for-service payment mechanism in wide use. Their aim was to provide all care, including preventive care and emotional support, using a payment-and-care delivery system that aimed to provide comprehensive care to a specific cohort of patients. The HMOs developed imaginative approaches to the high cost of care, including programs to prevent diseases and complications, programs to better manage chronic diseases, and methods to standardize care. They sought and incorporated clinical practice guidelines for the treatment of certain diseases, especially those such as asthma, diabetes, and heart failure that were particularly costly, and when no such guidelines were available, they developed their own. Capitation spread widely during the 1980s and 1990s. In some instances, this new delivery system reduced the cost of care quite remarkably, at least for a time.

But the new payment system soon found its detractors. Doctors were accused of withholding care to line their own wallets, and HMOs became even more severely reviled when they denied certain kinds of care such as bone-marrow transplants for advanced breast cancer (even though the effectiveness of the procedure had not been established scientifically) and were seen as hard-hearted and money-grubbing organizations. Ultimately, the health maintenance organizations lost a public relations battle over a handful of patients across the country who had been denied care (not always inappropriately), mostly by the for-profit organizations.

Many physicians expressed frustration in their capacity to deliver ideal care under HMOs, which frequently changed the drugs they were allowed to prescribe, second-guessed their clinical decisions, and challenged their autonomy. Financial incentives strained their professional principles. Competition had increased and technology demands strained their resources. Because their time was increasingly consumed by paperwork they viewed as valueless, by more and more meetings devoted to reporting requirements, and by the complex business activities forced on them, doctors had less time for personal activities. To maintain their incomes, many had to work longer hours and fit many more patients into their already-crowded schedules.[7]

Financing their practices became a major source of physicians' frustration. They found themselves in an increasingly competitive small business, and few had real business experience or special administrative acumen. Instead of the usual billing practices for one patient at a time, physicians had to negotiate contracts on an annual basis with not one, but many insurers. Practice management became an entirely new field involving competitive advantage, market share, negotiation, and cost accounting. And while the cost of care was increasing, insurers were reducing physicians' fees, sometimes abruptly and without warning. The cost of running doctors' offices increased as did the cost of malpractice insurance. All of these rising costs made physicians more attentive to the risks of their economic well-being and survival.

Physicians' incomes, which were high relative to the average worker, began to decline. Between 1995 and 1999 salaries and wages rose for most workers, but not for physicians. In that period, the average primary-care doctor's income, adjusted for inflation, fell by more than 6 percent; average specialists' income fell by 4 percent.[8] This decline almost certainly had an added effect on physicians' interest in compensating by finding other sources of income.

Yet it was not only money that discouraged doctors. They experienced frustrating payment delays, denials of claims, and increasingly complex and demanding regulations. Physicians whose bonuses depended on the number of referrals to subspecialists and on measures of productivity had higher levels of anxiety and concern that they might be compromising patient care than physicians whose bonuses were determined on the basis of the quality of care or of patient satisfaction. Some of the consequences of the dissatisfaction included early retirement, more disability filings, changes in careers, agitation about unionization, and quite recently, development of a new mode of practice called "concierge medicine": one that caters exclusively to wealthy patients. Regrettably, some physicians also began supplementing their incomes by distributing products such as vitamins, herbs, food supplements, cosmetics, and household cleaners, or by practicing the techniques of "alternative and complementary" medicine.

It's no wonder that doctors turned to sources of income other than patient care to maintain their standard of living. Cutbacks in reimbursement and increasing expenses, including malpractice insurance, put the squeeze not only doctors in medical centers but in community practice as well. One doctor in Pinole, California, is a case in point. He had always made a modest living and had not spent lavishly on material goods. He had always taken plenty of time with his patients, prided himself on the care he gave them, and was unwilling to compromise on the approach he learned long ago. Yet his pace of practice simply wasn't geared to sustaining even a reasonable income and before long he had to re-mortgage his home to pay his bills. A similar reaction from a physician in New England, who was financially unable to live in the community in which he practiced, shows how difficult many physicians have making ends meet from their practice income alone.

These assaults on physician autonomy and income and the new permissiveness that overlooks (and even accepts) financial conflicts of interest as part of political and business interactions contribute to a greater willingness of practicing physicians to engage in outside activities that can compromise their integrity, such as participating in the marketing efforts of drug companies, taking part in clinical trials run by for-profit research firms, purchasing drugs and selling them back to patients at a profit, or helping pharmaceutical companies to market their products. Such financial incentives have led to compromises in professional integrity.

Evolution of the Academic Physician

Changes in academic medicine in the past 50 years have been revolutionary. What started in mid-twentieth century as a modest, low-funded research activity dominated by a small cadre of academics with few, if any, ties with industry, has become a huge enterprise, with large fractions of research physicians in certain specialties co-opted by industry. Research in medicine changed largely because of new laboratory technology, but the attitudes of researchers about involvement with industry have undergone an equally radical evolution. The factors responsible for these attitudinal shifts were: a new federal law designed to enhance the economic power of the country through "technology transfer" from universities to industry, and an enormous infusion of money from the pharmaceutical, device, and biotechnology industries into clinical research. In addition, the remarkable growth in the number of researchers trained by NIH funding increased the cadre of academic researchers.

The perception of policy makers during the 1960s and 1970s was that there was a doctor shortage and that clinical research in the country was inadequate. Congress responded by providing the funding that allowed the NIH to increase the number of physicians in research fellowships. Some trained at the NIH, but many more trained in departments of academic medical centers around the country. There was no requirement after their research training to continue on in an investigative career. Many did so, but others went into private practice. As a consequence of the expansion of these specialty programs, clinical departments at medical centers around the country grew. By the early 1990s, divisions of departments of internal medicine, such as cardiology or gastroenterology had often grown to the size of their entire department only 10 to 15 years earlier. This growth in the number of researchers occurred as the pharmaceutical and medical-device industries poured large amounts of money into the coffers of the clinical departments for help in designing and implementing research on their products. The results of the enormous increase in investment in medicine by the government and industry were stunning. New drugs, new diagnostic tools, and new therapeutic devices came into being at an unprecedented pace.

A critical turning point came in 1974 when Harvard Medical School entered a 12-year agreement with Monsanto, a large chemical company with pharmaceutical products, which pledged $23 million in funding for construction of facilities to supply biological materials in return for an exclusive license for all inventions and discoveries made in connection with the project agreement. Historian Kenneth Ludmerer recently said: "The Monsanto-Harvard Medical School agreement was critical, in my view, in cultivating a new view that it was OK for medical schools to establish relationships with industry. In the 1950s and 1960s, HMS was donating its patents to the public. Now in the 1970s, with the new Monsanto agreement, HMS is allying itself with industry. And as Harvard does, most other U.S. medical schools do or try to do."[9] As it turned out, the Harvard-Monsanto agreement was a harbinger of remarkable changes to come.

Before 1980, only a small number of discoveries were converted into patents by universities; the Bayh-Dole Act changed this rate dramatically. Stimulated in part by the Harvard deal with Monsanto and the striking financial success of Stanford University (total royalties as of 2002, $255 million) in licensing recombinant cloning technology, many other universities not only developed their own patent offices but licensing and marketing capabilities as well.[10] By 1998 the number of patents produced by universities increased twentyfold, and businesses were "spun off" by faculty at an increasing rate. The financial incentives specified by the Bayh-Dole Act encouraged faculty members to disclose their inventions to the university, help prepare patent applications, and support the development and evaluation of resulting products. The university retains the patent, licenses it for a fee to one or more commercial enterprises, and industry then attempts to use the invention to develop profitable products.

At present, more than 100 universities and medical schools have invested in new companies to promote discoveries of their staff, and more than 150 institutions have "technology-transfer" offices.[11] In terms of profitability, however, the jury is still out on the value of patent and licensing offices to most of these institutions. Even though a new orientation toward a "business" strategy attracted more researchers into relations with industry, many academic medical centers have found it difficult to capitalize on the inventions and discoveries of their faculty. Though a few institutions generated windfall profits, most simply collected enough money from licensing agreements to fund their offices of technology transfer.[12]

One thing is quite clear: during the waning years of the twentieth century, many faculty members in the biosciences caught the rampant company-founding fever, with the approval of their academic institutions. Even relatively junior members of the Boston medical schools caught the shuttle to New York to consort with venture capitalists about their potentially profitable schemes.

During the mid-1960s, when NIH funding of research was growing, many researchers scorned others who had to appeal to pharmaceutical companies to support their work. Funding for research in infectious diseases, for example, was meager at that time, so researchers interested in these diseases often accepted industry funding for useful but not intellectually challenging antibiotic studies, and in doing so were able to squirrel away some of the leftover funds to support research projects that interested them more. As more new drugs were introduced in the 1980s, research support from industry grew and began to achieve more respectability. In 1980, however, Dr. Arnold Relman, then the editor in chief of the *New England Journal of Medicine*, sounded his first of several alarms at the possible adverse consequences of this collaboration.[13] Since then, industry support has exceeded NIH support by billions of dollars.[14]

By the late 1990s and to the present, procuring industry support for research has become the norm. Institutions now encourage young faculty members to seek such support not only to help fund their own salaries but to help fund research and clinical programs. In fact, given the large number of companies that many clinical investigators list when required to divulge their financial conflicts, I wonder whether there has been a gross turnaround in attitude among these researchers: the more companies for which they are consulting, the greater seems the admiration and respect of their colleagues.

Commercialization of Medicine Sets a New Tone

In the last two decades of the twentieth century, medicine joined many other disciplines that had already begun moving away from control by the government toward control in the private sector, including the utilities, the airlines, the telecommunications industry, and even to some extent, the military. Professional values, of course, are not etched in stone, but evolve in the context of the mores of the times. Given the remarkable conversion of the health-care system into a commercial enterprise since the early 1980s, physicians' perceptions about any competition between personal profits and patients' welfare became blurred.

In periods when NIH funding for research declined, medical school faculty members engaged more and more in the practice of medicine, fueled by reimbursements from Medicare and other insurers. At the time of enactment of Medicare in 1965 there were only approximately 17,000 full-time faculty members, but by 1990 their ranks had increased fivefold.[15] By the 1970s the academics were in heavy competition for patients with community physicians. By the 1980s, faculty emphasis on personal income had increased, and salaries increased sharply, made possible in part by enhanced income from medical practice. Faculty salaries, which had generally lagged behind those of community-based physicians, began to catch up and, in some instances, exceeded them. In some instances, those who billed for procedures on a fee-for-service basis (such as cardiologists and surgeons) were bringing in large amounts of revenue to their hospitals and were demanding and getting incomes of several hundred thousand dollars, and more.

Whereas some physicians in the community and in academia left practice or retired early; some, including academic physicians in medical centers, sensed the entrepreneurial and profit-making tone of the moment. This attitude exposed them to the new commercialism as well as a pervasive change in their role as professionals whose time-worn task was to put the patient first. Instead, they crossed the line and accepted profit making as an essential goal. As Dr. Kenneth Ludmerer said: "By the 1980s academic physicians were being compared with corporate executives, stockbrokers, and financial scoundrels in their greed and self-serving behavior."[16] Dr. Ludmerer's quote begins to capture the social environment of the past several decades, but there were further changes subsequently. In the mid 1990s, as the stock market boomed (and stocks of the pharmaceutical industry led the way), the country was intoxicated by commercialization. Our language reflected it: newspapers blazed with market values, return on investment, venture capital, and consumerism. (We even elected chief executive officers of corporations to be the leaders of our country.) And in medicine, while young physicians in training were working 100-hour weeks as house officers and earning $40,000 per year, their college roommates who went into law were being offered new positions at three to four times their medical friends' salaries, others in the securities business were making still higher multiples, and some of their friends in the dot-com world were already retiring. Young physicians saw their mentors in medicine becoming consultants for major drug companies, traveling around the world giving talks at resorts, and starting their own companies. Some physicians were away for weeks. Many who held back in making arrangements with pharmaceutical companies must have felt like suckers for not taking advantage of the opportunities that lucrative relations with industry presented.

Physicians, and especially their major organizations, lost substantial public trust. One index of this loss of trust was the virtual exclusion of physicians from the inner circle of planners involved in developing a national health-care plan in the early 1990s. Physicians were simply considered another special-interest group.[17]

The Current Climate

By the turn of the century, the big business bubble had begun to burst, but conflict of interest continued. I am reminded of a cartoon published in *USA Today* in July 2001, soon after Congress passed President Bush's tax rebate. Titled "Things You Can Buy with Your Tax Rebate Check. . . ." it depicts four items: a bicycle, a DVD player, clothes, and Your Congressman (shown ripping up a piece of paper containing the words "campaign re-form").[18] A politician's vote is one of the many things that money can buy. Needless to say, the pharmaceutical industry became one of the largest lob-bying groups.

The point is that physicians do not exist in isolation; rather, they are subject to changes in the culture and to the norms of society. And the norms of society, with respect to conflict of interest, have changed remarkably. In government, in the media, in the judicial system, in the securities business—to mention only a few—conflict of interest has become problematic, and despite occasional public outcries against blatant examples, serious con-flicts are often tolerated. Fresh in the minds of many are profit-motivated financial conflicts of interest that led to the demise of major corporations such as Enron and the accounting firm Arthur Andersen. But similar con-flicts are pervasive throughout society, and help to explain why they are tolerated in medicine. Here are few salient and well-known examples:

In 1999 Otis Chandler, the former owner of the *Los Angeles Times*, de-nounced the *Times'* new management for sharing profits with the Staples Center, a downtown sports arena, for a special weekend edition of the *Times Magazine* devoted exclusively to the new sports center.[19] In addition, the Staples Center had encouraged one of its suppliers to purchase advertising in the magazine. These financial agreements, among others, violated the traditional clear separation between editorial content and advertising.[20] To the credit of the newspaper's management, it ordered a full outside investigation and promised never to engage in such a conflict again.

In an interview with Matt Lauer in March 2002 on the *Today* show, Lauren Bacall urged people to get tested for macular degeneration, a vision-threatening disease that afflicted a friend. She mentioned that Visudyne, a new drug, could treat the disease, but neither she nor Matt Lauer indicated that she had been paid by the drug's manufacturer, Novartis, to mention the drug.[21] Ordinarily celebrities being paid by the pharmaceutical industry do not mention a specific drug: the drug companies' tactics are much more subtle. Instead, the entertainers are paid to appear in interviews to talk about a disease from which either they or one of their friends suffer; the audience is kept in the dark about the payments they receive. Rob Lowe, Danny Glover, and Kathleen Turner all have been paid participants in these campaigns by pharmaceutical manufacturers to heighten the awareness of diseases for which the companies have new (and often expensive) drugs.[22]

In an investigation that merited a Pulitzer Prize, *New York Times* reporter Gretchen Morgenstern uncovered several examples in which analysts and executives at investment banks sold their shares of companies while their analysts were issuing "buy" recommendations. In some cases, the stock lost 30 to 70 percent of its value after the analysts and executives sold off their own shares. Thus, the analysts, their executives, and their institutions benefited from inflated shares of the company's stock. Two notable examples involved Robertson Stephens, an international investment bank that focused on growth companies (now part of Fleet Bank). In September 2000, one of the Robertson Stephens stock analysts recommended that customers buy shares in iBasis, an Internet telephony provider, at the same time the analyst was selling more than 4,000 shares of the company's stock. In January 2001, another analyst for the bank continued to recommend a "buy" order on Corvis, a company that produced optical switching devices as Corvis' stock lost three-quarters of its value. The analyst continued to recommend that customers buy the stock even as he and company executives were selling shares worth more than a million dollars.[23]

Early in 2004, the *Wall Street Journal* published an expose on Edward D. Jones & Co., a brokerage partnership that had been recommending that investors purchase certain mutual funds.[24] Brokers are expected to make such recommendations on their perceived value of the funds, but in this case, almost all of Jones' sales of funds came from seven funds out of the 100 funds with which they had selling agreements. As it turned out, these seven funds had been paying Jones what was described as "hefty sums" in exchange for favoring the companies.

In government scientific advisory panels, the points of view of participants are required by law to be "fairly balanced," and the opinions of panelists are expected to be unimpeded by improper influences by special interests. In 1998, the General Accounting Office, at the request of Representative Henry A. Waxman (CA) audited several panels of scientists who advised the Environmental Protection Agency on regulations that govern toxic chemicals in the air and water supply. In one panel, 4 of the 13 members who assessed the carcinogenic potential of a chemical (1,3 butadiene, used in the manufacture of nylon and synthetic rubber) had worked for chemical companies or for industry-related research organizations. The panel recommended reclassifying the chemical from a "known" carcinogen to a "probable" carcinogen. In another panel responsible for assessing cancer risks, 7 of the 17 members had worked for similar organizations, and 5 other panel members had been paid consultants or received fees for other work from chemical companies.[25]

Abner Mikva, a former member of Congress and chief judge of the United States Court of Appeals for the District of Columbia, reported that between 1992 and 1998, more than 230 federal judges took trips to resorts to participate in seminars that were paid for by corporations or foundations that had an interest in curbing legislation on environmental protection, and that the judges might well be called on to participate in trials concerning such issues. Mikva described one judge who had attended a dozen trips by the three most prominent special interest groups.[26] Supreme Court Justice Antonin Scalia was widely criticized when he decided that he was capable of hearing an important case involving his friend Vice President Dick Cheney's refusal to disclose details of a White House energy task force. The reproach arose after Scalia's participation in January 2004 on duck-hunting trip with Cheney on the vice president's plane.[27] Allegations of possible bias erupted again when Chief Justice William Rehnquist appointed a committee on federal judicial ethics to review the practice of judges' acceptance of free vacations at resorts. Based on the previous actions of some members of the committee and the political connections of others, some wondered whether this particular committee would make sufficiently stringent recommendations.[28]

Texas, one of the few remaining states that elects its Supreme Court justices, has its share of complex conflicts. In 1997, lawyers or their firms and parties that had cases before the court gave 40 percent of the funds that the seven justices raised for their elections. In 1994, two months before a court ruling in a dispute about asbestos between American Petrofina and 55 other corporate defendants (on one side of a dispute) and local workers (on the other), Raul Gonzalez, one of the justices, took more than $84,000 in lawful campaign contributions from patrons of the corporations and defense lawyers.[29] The workers lost their case.

Because the Enron story exemplifies some of the worst conflicts of interest in business in recent years, it deserves more than passing mention. As is now widely known, Enron had created a series of partnerships and "related entities" with which it carried out well-hidden transactions. These partnerships made it possible to hide hundreds of millions of dollars in debt that the company's auditors either didn't see or intentionally overlooked. The chief financial officer of Enron, Andrew Fastow, must have known that Enron was in serious financial trouble, yet he continued to "manage outside partnerships that stood to profit from business dealings with Enron, in some cases putting Enron's assets at great risk" and to make millions of dollars himself from the partnerships as they slid deeper in debt.[30] These activities were described as an "extraordinary conflict of interest."[31] In addition, Enron executives sold $1.1 billion in their shares of stock before its stock price fell from approximately $85 per share to less than $1 per share. While the stock was tumbling, the auditors, Arthur Andersen, did not warn that the company was in serious financial straits. (In fact, Enron's third-quarter loss in 2001 was $618 million.) The chief executive, Kenneth Lay, was telling employees that the company was in good shape only days before disclosing a billion-dollar reduction in Enron's net worth. During that time Enron employees were prevented from selling the Enron shares in their retirement accounts, and many lost virtually their entire savings.[32] In December 2001, Enron filed for bankruptcy protection.

When Wendy L. Gramm, wife of former senator Phil Gramm, was head of the Commodities Futures Trading Commission in 1992, the commission exempted Enron's energy exchange business from government oversight. Senator Gramm was already receiving substantial campaign contributions from Enron at the time. Soon thereafter Wendy Gramm left the commission and was immediately appointed a paid director of Enron, and sat on the audit committee. Over the years she received more than a million dollars for her participation in Enron.[33] Also over the years, Senator Gramm received approximately $100,000 from Enron toward his elections. In 2000, Senator Gramm, who chaired the Senate Banking Committee, cosponsored a bill to deregulate some kinds of futures trading. When the bill became law, attached quietly to an 11,000-page appropriations bill, it allowed Enron to gain substantial control over electricity and natural gas. In 1998, Mrs. Gramm cashed in her Enron stock for more than $275,000 and continued to receive cash from Enron in a deferred account.[34] Thus she helped set the stage for enhanced Enron profits, then joined Enron. Senator Gramm's legislative actions further enhanced Enron's opportunities for profits while his wife continued as a paid member of Enron's board. As a member of Enron's audit committee, Mrs. Gramm was apparently unaware of Enron's questionable accounting that bankrupted the company. Senator Gramm profited both personally through his wife's actions and through substantial election financing. It seems that none of these shenanigans is illegal.

Needless to say, these are but a few examples of conflicts of interest in society at large, but they show how widespread they are and how emblematic they are in a social context.

Putting It Together

I have attempted to explain some of the factors that made many of America's doctors pay more attention to their own desires than to the health of their patients. I propose that the runaway cost of care, changing financial incentives, inflated income expectations, falling physicians' income, changes in patent law, and substantial influence of industry on medical research were essential ingredients. But societal and cultural factors also contributed heavily. Putting "business strategies" on a high pedestal encouraged many in medicine to ignore a long-held principle that the patient comes first, and a permissive attitude outside of medicine toward financial conflicts of interest, undoubtedly led many to think that such arrangements were also acceptable inside the walls of health care. The new complicity with industry spread like an infectious disease through a community. Many were immune to its invasiveness, but many were stricken.

The explanations for the cultural shifts in society that caused tumultuous changes in the ethics of business and decimated the savings of thousands of workers and retirees are beyond the scope of this work, but several factors have been cited. Corporate ethics have their ups and downs. In some eras speculation and greed take an upper hand until some of the perpetrators of schemes that benefited a few and injured many are exposed. In other eras, many corporate executives behaved as benevolent, public-spirited bureaucrats, running their companies with restraint and without rewarding themselves excessively for their efforts. Even in such circumstances the marketplace had a powerful influence, but it was counterbalanced by a code of ethics and a corporate culture that produced results that benefited society. In recent years a culture akin to greed gradually replaced one of restraint. (Interestingly, whereas the average chief executive officer of a Fortune 500 company earned 40 to 45 times the amount of the average salaried employee of the company in 1980, the multiple had increased tenfold by 2000.[35]) Unchecked market forces became the norm, and executives responded to the need for more profits and greater profit margins, sometimes introducing shady practices and even illegal transactions without regard for the general good of their employees or the country at large. Harvard professor Howard Gardner summed it up as follows, "How do people who want to do good work—work that is excellent and responsible—succeed or fail at a time when market forces are unprecedentedly powerful and there are no comparable countervailing forces?"[36]

We cannot guess today whether the reaction to these business disasters will trigger honest reform or whether we are in for more of the same. What we can say is that trust of the public in business leaders was badly shaken by the above revelations. Why is trust so important? Fundamentally, because major society functions depend on trust. Commenting on the accounting scandals of 2002, Charles Handy, in an article in the Harvard Business Review titled, "What's a Business For?" said, "Markets rely on rules and laws, but those rules and laws in turn depend on truth and trust. Conceal truth or erode trust, and the game becomes so unreliable that no one will want to play. The market will empty and share prices will collapse, as ordinary people find other places to put their money—into their houses, maybe, or under their beds."[37]

Trust in Medicine

The profession lost the public's trust when it was not accountable for the excesses of the fee-for-service payment system and when it did not speak out loudly enough against inappropriate restrictions of managed care. Many acted with disgust when newspaper and television stories documented examples of the free meals, trips to resorts, bonuses for enrolling patients in clinical trials, pseudoconsulting, and other financial deals. Such financial conflicts of interest have created an atmosphere of public distrust, and even though people generally trust their own physicians, the profession has lost some of its previous exalted position.

In fact, trust is the basis for the physician-patient relationship. I've not seen a better description of the covenant that must exist between a doctor and patient than one Cardinal Joseph Bernadin gave in a speech to the AMA. He explained that this covenant

> is grounded in the moral obligations that arise from the nature of the doctor-patient relationship. They are moral obligations—as opposed to legal or contractual obligations—because they are based on fundamental human concepts of right and wrong. While . . . it is not currently fashionable to think of medicine in terms of morality, morality is, in fact, the core of the doctor-patient relationship and the foundation of the medical profession.
>
> Why do I insist on a moral model as opposed to the economic and contractual models now in vogue? Allow me to describe four key aspects of medicine that give it a moral status and establish a covenantal relationship: First, the reliance of the patient on the doctor. Illness compels a patient to place his or her fate in the hands of a doctor. A patient relies,

not only on the technical competence of a doctor, but also on his or her moral compass, on the doctor's commitment to put the interests of the patient first. Second, the holistic character of medical decisions. A physician is a scientist and a clinician, but as a doctor is and must be more. A doctor is and must be a caretaker of the patient's person, integrating medical realities into the whole of the patient's life. A patient looks to his or her doctor as a professional adviser, a guide through some of life's most difficult journeys. Third, the social investment in medicine. The power of modern medicine—of each and every doctor—is the result of centuries of science, clinical trials, and public and private investments. Above all, medical science has succeeded because of the faith of people in medicine and in doctors. This faith creates a social debt and is the basis of medicine's call—its vocation—to serve the common good. Fourth, the personal commitments of doctors. The relationship with a patient creates an immediate, personal, non-transferable fiduciary responsibility to protect that patient's best interests. Regardless of markets, government programs, or network managers, patients depend on doctors for a personal commitment and for advocacy through an increasingly complex and impersonal system.

This moral center of the doctor-patient relationship is the very essence of being a doctor. It also defines the outlines of the covenant that exists between physicians and their patients, their profession, and their society. The covenant is a promise that the profession makes—a solemn promise—that it is and will remain true to its moral center. In individual terms, the covenant is the basis on which patients trust their doctors. In social terms, the covenant is the grounds for the public's continued respect and reliance on the profession of medicine.[38]

Patients must be able to trust their doctors. They should not have to be concerned that a doctor is recommending (or not recommending) a biopsy or a CT scan because the recommendation might be influenced by the doctor's financial arrangements. If they are asked to participate in a clinical trial, they should not have to wonder whether their participation is in the best interests of scientific medicine and not just in the best interests of their doctor.

We will never return to the perceived simple days of the past, but how much we trust and value doctors who care more for us than themselves is starkly illustrated by the exceptional amount of space that the *New York Times* devoted in 2002 to the obituary of "the $5 Doctor." In a four-column spread whose words reek of a lament for medicine as it was perceived to be in the past, the article lovingly described the life of Dr. Salvator Altchek, who had died at age 92 after practicing medicine in Brooklyn for 67 years. In more space than is typically devoted to the lives of widely acclaimed physicians, writers, and scientists, the writer quotes one of Dr. Altchek's patients as follows, "He wasn't out to make money; he was out to help people." The article mentioned that Dr. Altchek "generally attended to the health needs of anyone who showed up in his basement office in the Joralemon Street row house in the Heights where he lived, charging $5 or $10 when he charged at all." He "often made his house calls on foot, carrying his black medical bag. . . . For more than half a century, he began his workday at 8 A.M., took a half-hour off for dinner at 5 P.M., and closed the office door at 8. He then made house calls, often until midnight."[39]

A lot of newsprint for a simple family doctor, isn't it?

10

WHAT CAN BE DONE?

FINANCIAL CONFLICTS OF INTEREST THREATEN patient care, taint medical information, and raise costs. They create deception, impair physicians' judgment, and reduce their willingness to be their patients' advocates. They reduce professional dignity and integrity, denigrate the profession, and erode trust in the profession's practitioners, researchers, and institutions. To reverse the exceptional toll that financial conflicts exact will take some doing. We must start with principles.

Principles

Ideally, adherence to the highest professional creeds would be the best approach. Professionalism is a lofty ideal, but regrettably it lacks specificity and has not held sway as the onslaught of industry money has deflected many physicians' internal moral compasses. Whatever is done must be based on one assumption and four fundamental principles. The assumption, a solid one, is that gifts and financial entanglements, even minor ones, influence behavior and promote bias. The principles: First, financial considerations must never be allowed to compromise physicians' decisions about the care of individual patients or the safety of subjects involved in medical research. Second, because the integrity of scientific knowledge directly affects patient care, physicians' medical information must be free of bias generated by financial entanglements. Third, the profession must be accountable for insuring that undue commercial influence does not make the cost of care so high that it excludes many from receiving it. Last, we must aspire to the ideal of eliminating financial entanglements, but if physicians cannot or will not, we must have clear and enforceable methods that protect patients and complete disclosure about the conflicts. Though disclosure of financial arrangements is not an ideal solution, openness, honesty, and transparency about any financial arrangements is a minimum requirement.

The highest standard, and the one that would engender the most confidence, is elimination of financial conflicts of interest. Curiously, even some commercial organizations reach this standard. Lonely Planet Publications, publishers of travel books, makes the following statement in its books: "Lonely Planet books provide independent advice. Lonely Planet does not accept advertising in guidebooks, nor do we accept payment in exchange for listing or endorsing any place or business. Lonely Planet writers do not accept discounts or payments in exchange for positive coverage of any sort."[1]

And the wine writers for the *Wall Street Journal* described their policy as follows:

> For this column, we do not accept free wine, free trips, or free meals. We attend only events that are open to the public. We do not meet with winemakers when they visit New York. We buy all of our wines off retail shelves unless specifically noted otherwise. We shop, both in person and online, at retail stores all over the U.S., from Los Angeles to Chicago to Tallahassee, Fla. We taste wines blind unless noted otherwise. We believe wines should speak for themselves.[2]

Complete divestiture of all relations with industry may be the ideal, but I believe that it is unrealistic in the current political environment and because so much money is involved. Additionally, in some instances—for example, in creative and constructive scientific collaborations between physicians and industry—it could be counterproductive. I have no magic solutions to the heavy involvement of physicians with industry, but at the very least, all professional relations with industry must be based on the principles I described earlier, and they must be characterized by honesty, accountability, transparency, and openness.

Transparency Through Disclosure: Plusses and Minuses

Disclosing financial ties with industry is, by far, the most common means of dealing with conflicts in medicine. Disclosure operates under the principle that if financial conflicts of interest cannot or will not be eliminated, that transparency of the financial arrangements at least creates an informed recipient public. This "buyers-beware" approach assumes that individuals armed with disclosure information are able to judge whether the conflict might have or has had an influence; for example, whether information is biased. In fact, as shown by many examples throughout the book, it is difficult, and often impossible, for someone without highly specific expertise in a subject to identify a biased opinion in spoken or written material.[3] Disclosure of financial arrangements falters for other reasons. First, it is often ignored. Documents describing the conflicts may be systematically collected, but often left uninspected or unevaluated by authorities. Even when such information is collected, it is often not available to the public. The FDA regulations governing the conflicts of interest for investigational new drug applicants, for example, require disclosure to institutional review boards and to the FDA itself, but not to study subjects or to the broader public.[4] In this sense, disclosure is not really made, nor is it truly public.

There are many serious flaws with policies that rely on disclosure.[5] Disclosure requires people to assess a person's motives and guess whether his actions may have been affected by any conflicts. They may assume, incorrectly, that a financial conflict is evidence at face value that an individual is incapable of producing unbiased information. In fact, some believe that disclosing financial conflicts serves only to call unnecessary attention to a problem that may not exist, and at its worst is simply accusatory. They worry that disclosing such conflicts may reduce the public's confidence in the validity of medical advice and research. In fact, even though disclosure is intended to bolster public confidence, it may actually undercut it.

Further, disclosure can be observed to the letter while avoiding the intent. When lecturers flash their financial arrangements on a few quick slides or leave the list on a desk outside a lecture hall, for all practical purposes the information is unavailable. (The American Society of Hematology, in its 2000 annual meeting wins the prize for obscurity. In the program of the meeting it simply listed the numbers of the presentations in which an author disclosed a financial conflict of interest. No indication is given what the conflicts were.)[6] A major problem is that only naming a company provides limited information because it fails to specify which drugs or devices the company manufactures. Because not all participants in the meeting are intimately familiar with the relevant products of each declared company, they may be unaware of a potential for bias.

Moreover, a standard definition of financial conflict has yet to be established throughout the medical community, which renders so-called disclosure meaningless. Of course, because declarations are voluntary, the accuracy of individual declarations is not verified. And even when all members have disclosed their financial conflicts, members of the panel may not remember who had specific conflicts when a particular drug or device is being discussed. Further, nobody wants to be an accuser: even when a committee member perceives that a bias might exist in one or more members' opinions, the sensitivity of an accusation of bias is often so great he is likely to be too embarrassed to speak up. Just as nobody wants to insult his host at a dinner party, few people are willing to challenge their colleagues' motives openly. The net effect of all these reservations is that open disclosure is of extremely limited value.

In fact, it may be much worse than I have indicated. Disclosure in educational settings and in clinical-guideline committees may have the effect of sanitizing the entire proceeding. Such perfunctory disclosures may give a quiet nod to a conflicted participant, thus giving him a license to make any recommendation, no matter how biased. George Loewenstein, an economics professor at Carnegie Mellon University, identifies similar problems with disclosure in the business world. He said, "If you disclose a conflict of interest, people in general don't know how to use that information. . . . And to the extent that they do anything at all, they actually underestimate the severity of these conflicts." Commenting on the response of observers who had been told about an individual's conflict of interest, Lowenstein said, "You know the score, so now anything goes. People are grasping at the straw of disclosure because it allows them to have their cake and eat it too."[7] Reporter James Surowiecki adds, "It has become a truism on Wall Street that conflicts of interest are unavoidable. In fact, most of them only seem so, because avoiding them makes it harder to get rich. That's why full disclosure is so popular: it requires no substantive change."[8]

Only a select few institutional policies that rely on disclosure actually specify to whom the disclosure must be made (for example, to institutional review boards, other institutional bodies, funding agencies, or the government), and of these, even fewer mandate disclosure to patients or the public. Institutions also get lazy when they can just point to their disclosure policy but have no monitoring mechanism. Such "window dressing" serves little purpose. It is a fallacy that something about disclosing, or public "confession" of financial conflicts magically "eliminates" bias, as though somehow it operates directly on the individual's psyche. When we announce our conflicts, we quietly and symbolically wink at each other that objectivity reigns. Instead, disclosure has come to be treated as a formality, just another piece of paper to fill out, rather than a solemn moment during which people take inventory of their integrity.

Although disclosure is not a particularly high standard, and has flaws, it is better than no disclosure at all. But disclosures must include the amounts of money physicians receive for their services and must name the specific products that might come under question because of the financial ties.[9] Just naming the company that makes the product is not sufficient.

Policies of Our Professional Organizations

How do the policies of major medical organizations stack up against the assumption and the four principles of professionalism previously described? I think not very well, in part because they disregard the notion that gifts influence behavior. According to the American Medical Association (AMA) policies, gifts are allowed, but should "primarily entail a benefit to patients and should not be of substantial value." Dinners should be "modest meals." Social events should have only a modest value to the physician; they should facilitate discussion among attendees. Subsidies from industry should not be accepted "to pay for the costs of travel, lodging, or other personal expenses of physicians attending conferences or meetings. . . . There can be no link between prescribing or referring patterns and gifts."[10] Thus the AMA expects individual physicians to decide whether an event in which they are asked to participate "entails a benefit" to patients and to interpret the meaning of "substantial value" and "modest value." Needless to say, there is considerable latitude in such interpretations. The AMA publicizes its policy (supported, of course, by industry) but does not monitor compliance.

The policies of another influential organization, the American College of Physicians (ACP) are based on physicians' willingness to examine their own practices and judge their acceptability based on whether they would be willing to have them known to the public. They state, "the acceptance of even small gifts has been documented to affect clinical judgment and heightens the perception (as well as the reality) of a conflict of interest. While following the Royal College of Physicians' guideline [also known as the *New York Times* test], 'Would I be willing to have this arrangement generally known?' physicians should also ask, 'What would the public or my patients think of this arrangement?'"[11] There is an inconsistency in this policy. If even small gifts are problematic, then why be concerned with the appearance of any "arrangements"? Why not simply proscribe gifts? Moreover, the "Royal College of Physicians" and the *New York Times* tests (the widely known standards) fail: first, because many physicians do not even appreciate that gifts of various kinds can influence their behavior, and second, because embarrassment is a highly variable attribute. Some physicians are embarrassed to take even a pen, a pad of paper, or a textbook. Others—perhaps the thick skinned or arrogant—would not be ashamed no matter who found out about their sponsored trips to resorts or their paid efforts on the part of industry. Some even brag about their "take."

Other groups and individuals have weighed in on physicians' responsibilities. As part of a collaborative project of the American Board of Internal Medicine, the American College of Physicians, and the European Federation of Internal Medicine, their *Charter on Medical Professionalism* includes "Commitment to maintaining trust by managing conflicts of interest" as one of its ten professional responsibilities. Its conflict-of-interest provision differs little from existing guidelines, mostly because it adheres to the "disclosure" model of conflict management. It says, "Physicians have an obligation to recognize, disclose to the general public, and deal with conflicts of interest that arise in the course of their professional duties and activities. Relationships between industry and opinion leaders should be disclosed, especially when the latter determine the criteria for conducting and reporting clinical trials, writing editorials or therapeutic guidelines, or serving as editors of scientific journals."[12] Nonetheless, this policy does recommend disclosure to the "general public," including patients, a constituency that is rarely recognized explicitly in other guidelines. Unfortunately, the action "deal with" is vague.

All of these guides to professional behavior regarding financial conflict of interest are worthy, yet they contain too many "shoulds," not enough "musts," and are fundamentally unenforceable. Also, the existing AMA and ACP policies largely ignore other more serious conflicts, namely consulting arrangements, speaker's bureaus, and production of educational materials. No member of the American College of Physicians has been expelled because of an undisclosed financial conflict of interest. It seems quite likely that this is true of most other organizations as well.

In fact, other professions have far more stringent guidelines and rules from which medical organizations can learn.

Comparative Conflict-of-Interest Guidelines

Lawyers are subject to several layers of regulation and oversight by the American Bar Association (ABA), state bar associations, judicial review boards, strong professional norms, firm self-policing, background checks, and vigilant court officers. According to the *Model Rules of Professional Conduct,* "a judge should disqualify himself or herself in a proceeding in which the judge's impartiality might reasonably be questioned."[13] If an attorney becomes aware of a conflict of interest that impairs his ability to represent a client, he is obligated to ask the client to find another attorney. Lawyers in violation of such professional canons face a variety of sanctions, ranging from dismissal of a case to disbarment. The adversarial court system is a potent influence in reducing the chance of serious conflicts. If an attorney in a case discovers a financial conflict of interest in an opposing lawyer, he can bring it to the attention of the court.

In medicine no such adversarial situation exists, but physicians' reputations are dear to them. Because financial conflicts are largely hidden, however, nobody can be embarrassed now by their arrangements with one more company. All the more reason to make the financial ties between physicians and industry public knowledge.

The United States Constitution regulates conflicts of interest among government employees.[14] Because government agents are considered public trustees, they are held to particularly high standards. The laws primarily prohibit the formation of conflictive relationships but also punish misconduct.[15] Members of Congress and their staffs and former officials are prohibited, for example, from helping private parties negotiate favorable treatment from the government.[16] Regulations are enforced by regular audits by the Office for Government Ethics, and by ethics officers within regions and buildings of every government office. It is important to note, however, that some federal officials have the capacity to waive the restrictions under certain circumstances.

Compliance with conflict-of-interest policies among federal government employees is based on "good faith," but the measures are backed by active policing and sanctions. Sanctions include advisory opinions, warnings, orders to divest, loss of committee assignment, civil monetary penalties, impeachment, and referral to the attorney general.

In medicine there is little policing and virtually no sanctions for physicians with financial conflicts. Professional organizations must no longer look away from this issue. If they wish to retain the trust of the public, they must develop far more high-minded policies, indeed ones that would embarrass physicians who collaborate with industry's marketing goals and would reward doctors who keep free of such conflicts. I challenge the ACP and AMA and other major professional organizations to upgrade the standards for their members and show the public that they intend to take a much higher ground on the issue of conflict of interest.

The ethical responsibilities of journalists are bound up more in a "covenant with society" than with any body of regulation. Both professional journalism associations and individual news companies have ethical codes, which typically include conflicts of interest among their prohibited behaviors. Decisions are often made on several levels, from the individual reporter to the desk editor to the publisher, and are subject to ever-shifting factors such as political climate. Ethical trespasses have often been dealt with on a case-by-case basis within individual news organizations.[17]

As with lawyers, the most effective enforcement mechanism may be the intense public scrutiny borne by reporters as a direct consequence of the visibility of their work. Reporters competing for news stories often follow one another's leads, and thus place checks on one another. Source citing is subject to intense scrutiny, especially within reputable news organizations. Reporters are expected to recuse themselves from covering material that would expose an overt personal bias.

The *New York Times* sweeping new conflict-of-interest policy "Ethical Journalism: Code of Conduct for the News and Editorial Departments," a major development in journalistic ethics, governs the relationship between the private lives of reporters and officials and their journalistic pursuits. The provisions cover not only financial conflicts of interest, but also political and civic participation, plagiarism, relationships to sources, the paper's neutrality, intellectual property, and the behavior of family members. Among its provisions:

> No staff member may own stock or have any other financial interest in a company, enterprise or industry the coverage of which he or she regularly provides, edits, packages or supervises or is likely regularly to provide, edit, package or supervise. A book editor for example, may not invest in a publishing house, a health writer in a pharmaceutical company or a Pentagon reporter in a mutual fund specializing in defense stocks. For this purpose industry is defined broadly; for example, a reporter responsible for any segment of media coverage may not own media stock. "Stock" should be read to include futures, options, rights, and speculative debt, as well as "sector" mutual funds (those focused on one industry).[18]

Why should the guidelines for reporters be far more stringent than those for doctors? Isn't a doctor's covenant with society just as meaningful and important? That physicians are not held to the standards of journalists, attorneys, and other professionals is one of the great scandals of our time. In contrast to the rules and guidelines that govern other professionals, those that govern medicine are missing: proscription against investments in drugs they recommend, mandatory disclosure of all conflicts (naming specific drugs, devices, and dollar amounts), openness to public scrutiny, elimination of major commercial entanglements, and strict governmental regulation.

The Status of Regulation

Free markets can work well as long as government stands ready to limit their excesses. In the last several years some states have begun to take an active role in financial conflicts of physicians, but these efforts were spurred by rising drug costs, not by ethical issues. Vermont passed a law regulating the disclosure of gifts from pharmaceutical companies to doctors.[19] The law does not forbid gifts, but requires that pharmaceutical companies (not doctors) report any gifts to physicians greater than $25 in value (including honoraria and travel costs), other than drug samples. The state plans to post the disclosures on the Internet as an incentive for doctors not to take the gifts.[20] Governor Howard Dean, a physician himself, said, "I do think doctors are swayed."[21] No disclosures are anticipated in Vermont until late in 2004. California and several other states are considering similar bills, but because all of these efforts focus narrowly on gifts and travel, they miss the far more subtle, long-lasting, and pervasive types of financial interest, such as consulting relationships, royalty and licensing agreements, stock ownership, positions on corporate boards, and marketing efforts that are cloaked as research. In addition, pharmaceutical companies can easily maneuver around these cursory requirements, and are likely to continue to engage physicians by simply restructuring the income transfer and calling it something other than a gift.

After the revelations in the criminal case involving TAP Pharmaceuticals, the office of the United States inspector general (OIG) began to consider whether pharmaceutical gift giving might qualify under federal "fraud and abuse" policies. After issuing broad guidelines for the pharmaceutical industry in draft form, the OIG backed off somewhat, in part because of strong lobbying by both the pharmaceutical industry and the AMA. Both groups sought to retain physicians' ability to receive "modest" gifts, consult for industry, and partake in industry-sponsored CME activities.[22] The final OIG guidance preserves almost all of the activities requested by industry and the AMA, and more or less reflects both AMA and new PhRMA guidelines. But it strengthens the proscription against some of the worst practices ("shadowing," for example), and it has placed physicians at risk of federal action if they combine a financial arrangement with an agreement to fund an educational program, or if they engage in pseudoconsulting.[23] Physicians will have to be wary of crossing the line. In deciding whether a given action might be in violation of federal kickback laws (the Anti-Kickback Act of 1970), the OIG said it would assess actions based on these questions:

does the practice compromise clinical judgment? is information provided accurate and complete? could the arrangement increase government costs? and could the arrangement lead to inappropriate utilization of health-care resources?

What More Is Needed?

I believe that proscriptions against financial conflicts have not gone far enough. Sometimes government must step in when markets usurp too much power, and when social problems get out of control. It has done so in many spheres including unemployment compensation, retirement benefits, and medical care for the elderly. If the profession cannot be more accountable by its independent actions, government must intervene. It would be relatively easy to compel physicians and organizations (virtually all of whom receive federal funds in one form or another) to comply with more stringent conflict-of-interest regulations. I hope such intervention will not be necessary because regulations are likely to be heavy-handed and lack the nuances to preserve the benefits of physician-industry collaboration. In fact, opposition to more governmental regulations is likely to be fierce: the AMA has traditionally fought them, and the vast lobbying resources of the pharmaceutical and biotechnology industries would undoubtedly be used to block any attempt to limit industry ties to physicians. Finally, the political climate for any such intervention is notably unfavorable.

There is no simple way to preserve the entrepreneurial spirit that has created MRI scans, stents, bioengineered drugs, and artificial knees and at the same time completely eliminate financial conflicts of interest. The practice of researchers' developing products and testing them in their own institutions, especially on their own patients, is the most serious issue, and there may be no perfect approach when this problem arises. The American Society of Gene Therapy restricts investigators from enrolling patients, managing a study, or obtaining informed consent from patients in a clinical trial that is sponsored by a private company in which they hold an equity interest. A member that violates this rule can be expelled from the organization.[24] The new Harvard Medical School rules contain a similar proscription, and in the interest of patient safety, I believe this action is justified.

Some believe, however, that this policy is too restrictive. Guidelines by the AAMC allow investigators to carry out clinical research on their own inventions only when no other researcher could reasonably do the study.[25] New federal guidelines also make such an allowance, but require stringent independent oversight to insure that the research is likely to benefit patients and that study participants are not subjected to undue risk.[26] Failing a complete proscription of clinical research by financially conflicted investigators, institutions must invite a substantial membership of lay people to be members of the groups that make decisions in which such conflicts are considered. They should cede their decision-making autonomy on this issue to an outside, independent group, perhaps retaining a minority membership, or appoint an ombudsman with independent power to block any work that is considered inappropriate.[27] All of these oversight methods could also be used in circumstances other than research to protect patients and to reduce bias in medical information when financial conflicts have not been completely eliminated.

If we expose medical schools and academic medical centers that offer CME credits for courses in which they have little involvement in organizing or running, perhaps they will stop doing so. If industry funds continue to flow into physicians' education, the influence of such sponsorship can never be eliminated entirely: someone is always going to know which company sponsored the programs and could potentially be influenced by the arrangement. But safeguards can be built in. CME departments must reject industry sponsorship unless they control faculty choices and program content. Companies must not be asked to nominate participants just because they supply the funds, and any faculty chosen must have no financial stake in a course's content. The point is that industry support of physicians' education must have no strings attached. (Because such unencumbered educational grants were given in the past, and because the companies have an enormous incentive to be liked by physicians, I believe there would be little lapse in the provision of such funds.) Institutions must seek many more educational funds in the form of endowed lectureships; departments must be aggressive about finding funds to pay for the education of their members that are not dependent on industry.

Professional organizations should eliminate drug-company-sponsored "symposia" during their major medical meetings. They should stop cooperating with the companies in sending out their brochures, offering them their membership and conference participant lists, and accepting payments for these services. Professional organizations should disallow all lectures by physicians in the display areas of their meetings. They must also stop accepting funds for tasks that could directly benefit industrial partners; financial support from industry must be unencumbered by direct expectations of reciprocity. Company prizes and travel awards, which can have a great positive impact on young investigators, must require no quid pro quo. Drug company advertising must have no direct relation to content on professional society publications.

The quality of the pharmaceutical industry's products should speak for itself, without requiring massive marketing to physicians or marketing by physicians. The pharmaceutical industry has argued that its huge expenditures for marketing to doctors is directed mainly at educating physicians. If that is truly their goal, I challenge them to contribute to a pool of educational funds that could be parceled out by an independent body in some equitable fashion. Contributors to such a fund would be recognized for their participation. This suggestion was not rejected out of hand when I suggested it to a senior executive of PhRMA.[28] Surely, such a plan would be complex, but it is not an impossible dream. The pharmaceutical industry should want to avoid even the perception that its marketing efforts are tainting the very profession on which it depends for its success.

The process of clinical-practice-guideline development requires special attention because it has such an enormous impact on the quality of patient care. We must end the practice of perfunctory disclosures followed by business as usual. We must admit that the usual approach to announcing conflicts is often a sham. Some say that because so many of the top academic physicians are involved with industry, they could never find enough people with sufficient expertise to deal with the complexities of the clinical problem. I call this the "fallacy of unique expertise." I admit that when a product is brand new and no one else has expertise, perhaps the only ones with sufficient knowledge might be one or two experts. In such instances, we may have no choice but to listen to their judgments about the products. Nonetheless, this should be an unusual case: often many others quickly develop expertise, and conflicted experts will not be needed to develop practice guidelines.

I have often been told that only those "close to the action," that is, those with industry ties, have sufficient expertise to develop such guidelines (some journal editors say the same about recruiting authors to write editorials), yet nobody has provided any evidence that people with financial ties to industry are better in assessing evidence on any a particular subject than those without such ties. Large cadres of clinicians are engaged in systematic evaluation of evidence ("evidence-based medicine"), and clinicians use the assessments of these panels all the time. There is no fundamental reason to think that such panels of intelligent clinicians who have no industry connections would be unable to assess a body of clinical data and arrive at useful recommendations.

In fact, there is real risk that like-minded people with "unique" knowledge may have similarities of thought and come up with a uniform conclusion that is biased (or even completely wrong). They may be subject to what the military calls "incestuous amplification," which *Jane's Defense Weekly* defines as "a condition in warfare where one only listens to those who are already in lock-step agreement, reinforcing set beliefs and creating a situation ripe for miscalculation."[29] Even some people in highest authority fail to appreciate how misleading such insular advice can be.[30]

Even though a great many experts are conflicted, there are ways to lessen the chance of bias in clinical-practice-guideline development. Participation on these guideline committees is a prestigious appointment. One choice is to save such "prizes" for those with no financial ties, that is, to reward people who stay free of personal financial entanglements with industry. (Journal editors could do the same when they recruit people to write editorials and review articles, but at present few do.) If we did this, we would undoubtedly lose the services of some talented people who have decided to accept personal funds from industry, but that would be the price we would have to pay for trying to avoid bias. Another choice is to allow only a small minority of physicians who have financial conflicts to serve on clinical-practice-guideline committees. A third choice is to engage neutral people who know the full details of conflict-of-interest disclosures (including dollar amounts) to rigorously screen all candidates for service on practice-guideline committees and exclude those who they believe are at high risk of professional compromise. Minority reports should be regularly allowed and published along with the full report.

Government intervention is also warranted on industry-initiated and industry-sponsored "front organizations." These groups, often led by financially conflicted physicians, sponsor ventures such as pamphlets, brochures, pocket books, Web sites, and registries, and they have gotten out of hand, often subtly recommending off-label drugs and promoting expensive drugs. Although federal agencies have control over drug advertising, these ventures apparently have escaped detection and oversight. Nonetheless, they may have even more impact on the use and misuse of drugs than pharmaceutical advertising in medical journals and in the lay media. These publications masquerade as educational materials, but many are largely marketing efforts that deserve as much scrutiny as drug advertisements.

Based on the principles of honesty and openness, any remaining financial conflicts must be available for public scrutiny. To make it easier for physicians and consumers to identify the physicians who have financial arrangements, a mechanism must be found, perhaps under the leadership of the AAMC, for hospitals, health centers, and academic medical centers, to contribute regularly to a voluntary, searchable Web-based registry of faculty members and associated physicians who have financial conflicts of interest. Such a registry could include those on pharmaceutical company boards, advisory committees, speaker's bureaus, and recipients of grants. Names could remain from the time that the relationship begins and for two years thereafter. I recognize that such a list might only contribute to an existing culture of popularity and stature of conflicted physicians, yet it would be much easier with such a registry to identify who has the conflicts and how the conflict might have played out. I can also anticipate objections on the basis of privacy, yet there is already a precedent for such widespread disclosures: they are already required on many educational materials and by many journals. Universal Web-based disclosure is an idea worthy of further consideration.

Teaching about the effects of conflict of interest must start as students first walk through the doors of the medical schools, and it must be reinforced every year thereafter. Nearly all schools have courses in medical ethics, but conflict of interest is not a consistent part of these curricula. Needless to say, the schools may find proscription of gifts and meals difficult to justify if their faculty are heavily involved with industry themselves. Students should be encouraged not to take gifts or interact with drug salesmen. House staff should pay for meals themselves rather than be obligated to drug sales-men and their companies. House officers must be encouraged not to meet with drug salesmen outside their institutions. Only a few medical schools and training programs proscribe companies from providing free food and gifts, but those that do make an important statement to their students and trainees about professionalism.

Toward a Higher Standard

Several people have written that physicians should say no to most industry collaborations[31] and many efforts have been made to reconfigure medicine's approach to conflicts of interest.[32] Each of the latter consists of an attempt to clarify the norms and values on which medicine is based as well as pro-posals for procedures that could accomplish the profession's ideal goals. They have some of the right characteristics, including sponsorship by promi-nent, high-minded, ethical individuals. Unfortunately, these pronounce-ments leave the enforcement to local organizations. Not one powerful medical center has declared war on financial conflicts. None has outlawed faculty participation in speaker's bureaus, participation in consulting ar-rangements that are thinly veiled marketing efforts, or completely elimi-nated company-sponsored meals. Many set no limits on stock options or income from patent royalties. Most have no rules about how often their faculty members can be involved with for-profit entities. And the rules that most institutions do invoke are often enforced irregularly. Few institutions have turned their conflict-of-interest issues over to a regulative body that is independent of the parent institution, but that is exactly what they should do. I have suggested various oversight mechanisms for research and for com-mittee deliberations, and they would work equally well for institutional rules.

In the end, medical care cannot be treated exclusively as a commodity. We must provide safeguards to protect the public as medicine becomes inextricably bound to industry. Patients have the right to disinterested pro-fessional judgment. As I have asserted before, it shouldn't have to be pa-tients' responsibilities to protect themselves against the medical profession. Even with rigorous guidelines, pharmaceutical companies will seek ways to influence physicians, especially prominent academics and community "thought leaders." Doctors must take personal responsibility for their behavior. Leading clinicians will have to refuse to be paid consultants. Though many will deny it, it is too easy to be seduced to favor one company over another or to prescribe a particular drug when one company is indirectly paying your daughter's college tuition. Individual physicians will have to refuse meals, gifts, books, pens, and tote bags with company labels, invitations to join speaker's bureaus, and consulting arrangements other than those for scientific purposes.

What do we say to others who are not so sure of where they stand? We can apply Howard Gardner's "mirror test." We can ask them to try to perceive themselves as accurately as possible, perhaps with the help of critical colleagues, when they answer these questions: "When you think of yourself as a professional, are you proud or ashamed? When you think of your fellow professionals, are you proud or ashamed, and if the latter, what are you prepared to do about it?"

The societal gift of professional autonomy requires that each physician act responsibly, contribute to a culture of integrity, and help develop the means of self-monitoring. All physicians must be encouraged to assess whether they are capable of developing financial relationships with industry without compromising their integrity. Such introspection must get at difficult personal questions, including whether they could allow the quest for personal wealth to compromise medical education, medical research, patient care, and the information on which such care depends. Physicians must know their institutional or professional society ethical guidelines and work to improve them when they are lax. Such guidelines must not be treated as a maximum allowable restraint, but as a minimum code of conduct. Physicians must not forget that they are important societal role models, and that how they act will determine what the profession is and will become. For those who follow them—the students and house officers—they must show that greed and entrepreneurialism is neither a necessary nor desirable cultural attribute.

What Can the Public Do?

The public must become involved if we are to change the greed culture that permeates medicine. What is needed is a sustained public outcry against inappropriate practices. My hope is that readers of this book will demand that members of Congress who have launched narrow investigations into financial conflicts in medicine widen their inquiries. They could ask Congress to request studies of the problem by the distinguished Institute of Medicine in Washington in the same depth as the institute did for patient safety and medical errors. They could also pressure Congress to reassess the risks and benefits of the provision in the Bayh-Dole act that cedes huge royalties to investigators. I urge trustees of medical organizations to examine the conflict-of-interest guidelines of their own institutions, make sure that they exist, have enforcement mechanisms, and are updated. There will be a tendency to rewrite them so that they are only in compliance with the OIG guidance, but they could do much more: the foregoing principles and goals can show how.

Many talented journalists have repeatedly uncovered some of the worst conflicts and their worst outcomes, but often the stories are seen as isolated events. A "fix" is applied, and then we wait until the next time. To insure that these stories have lasting effects, people must come forth to demand reform in the medical profession, demand that the extensive interlocking of physicians with industry be modulated, and that physicians must be the implements of change.

The public must demand that physicians with special responsibilities, including senior officials of health-care institutions, officers of professional organizations, editors of medical journals (associate and deputy editors as well), panelists at the FDA, scientists at the NIH, principal investigators of large clinical studies, and heads of clinical-practice-guideline committees have no financial conflicts. These posts must be considered prestigious prizes to be reserved for the nonconflicted. The public must call for full disclosure of the financial arrangements between professional organizations and industry.

Swimming Against the Current

Fifteen years ago when Dr. Stephen Goldfinger of Harvard Medical School warned about the increasing acceptance of industry largesse, one critic of his commentary said: "At best, Dr. Goldfinger's comments appear naïve; at worst, they smack of a holier-than-thou moralism that harks back to a bygone era.

Times are changing, and we should not be like the dinosaurs, who at their last board meeting before extinction uniformly voted not to change. The pharmaceutical industry is not the Evil Empire. It is an equal partner in the health care endeavor, and we could improve matters substantially by encouraging a more equal partnership with it."[33] I don't know whether the commentator still believes that the drug industry is an equal partner, but I do know that drug companies have so infiltrated medicine that few physicians are untouched by their tentacles.

Is it realistic to think that the extensive involvement by physicians with industry can be reduced? Physicians' self-image and their dedication to a high standard of professionalism are the only influences that deter them from industry entanglements. Unfortunately, all the principal incentives are powerful countervailing forces, and without intense public pressure, the pharmaceutical industry will continue to devote enormous resources to engaging physicians, academic institutions, and professional organizations in marketing efforts. The professional societies seem to be unwilling to confront their members with tough regulations, and the academic medical centers seem frightened that if they do so, their best scientists will go elsewhere.

Despite the continued slide toward more industry involvement, several experiences leave me some encouragement. The publication committee of the American Heart Association made the absence of financial conflicts of interest a prerequisite for editorship of its flagship journal. And the Endocrine Society was far more careful and conservative in its recommendations for a second generation of practice guidelines on screening for thyroid disease. The resistance of some medical organizations such as the Society of General Internal Medicine, the American College of Psychiatry, the Group for the Advancement of Psychiatry, the American Society of Clinical Oncology, and the American Society of Gene Therapy to commercial ties is another positive sign. And at its 2002 annual meeting, the American Medical Student Association departed from the AMA and approved a policy that urges physicians, residents, and students not to accept gifts from the pharmaceutical industry, urges hospitals to stop pharmaceutical company-funded lectures and lunches on- and off-site, urges physicians not to accept honoraria from industry for speaking and for token consulting, and opposes giving CME credit for drug-company-sponsored events.[34]

A Possible Roadmap

Items for immediate implementation:

1. Exclusion of *all* gifts from industry (by law if necessary), even including items that might be considered useful in a doctor's practice or education; elimination of physician participation in company-sponsored speaker's bureaus.

2. Prohibition of consultations with industry for anything except scientific matters, and outlawing of marketing by physicians of drugs or devices in which they have a financial interest.

3. Full disclosure to patients in all doctors' private offices of any and all financial incentives for patient care or clinical research.

4. Elimination of "finder's fees" for identifying patients to drug companies or their intermediates; no "farming out" of patients for clinical research.

5. Permission to conduct clinical research on devices or drugs in which the investigator has a financial interest should be proscribed.

6. The requirement of full accessibility for independent analysis of all data in any published clinical trial in which the investigators had a financial conflict.

7. A requirement of full, detailed disclosure in legible handouts at all teaching events of the type (drugs or devices), dollar amounts, and duration of all financial ties of the lecturer that relate to the subject at hand; full disclosure of the sponsorship of all such events.

8. The selection of journal editors, officers of major professional organizations, and leaders of academic institutions among physicians who have no financial conflicts.

9. A demand for increased scrutiny by medical editors of all financial conflicts of authors, with full disclosure not only of the company relationships but also the specific relevancy of the conflicts to the subject matter (specific drugs and devices).

10. Pressure for a comprehensive analysis of the problem by the Institute of Medicine that would include drafting principles and guidelines for all types of financial conflicts, not just those associated with research.

Items for further analysis and debate:

1. If CME lectures by individuals with financial conflicts cannot be prohibited, should physicians boycott courses given by financially conflicted lecturers?

2. If clinical-practice-guideline committees cannot be constituted exclusively by nonconflicted individuals, what safeguards can be introduced to reduce the chance of biased recommendations?

3. If ownership of stock in a company that could benefit from a researcher's work and scientific consultations with a company create conflicts, what is the basis for any specific "minimally acceptable" amount that researchers can hold in stock or receive yearly in compensation for consultations?

4. How could a universal Web-based registry of physicians' financial conflicts of interest be implemented?

5. How can the financial arrangements of professional organizations with industry be disclosed, including the amounts, duration, and purposes for which the funds were used?

6. How can the dependence of professional organizations on industry support be reduced?

7. Can industry be convinced that in the long run the harm of physicians' collusion with their marketing practices is more serious than the short-term gain in sales?

None of these questions will be addressed without strong pressure of the public and the avid participation of leaders of professional organizations and academic medicine. I challenge them to take up the battle.

Most physicians think of a career in medicine as a calling, and practice the principle they agreed to when they joined the profession, namely to "come for the benefit of the sick, remaining free of all intentional injustice [and] of all mischief." Nonetheless, as we have seen, the line between true professionalism and overt exploitation can be indistinct: collaborating with industry can benefit patient care, but at the same time it can bias physicians' actions. Though an individual's motives may be difficult for an outsider to fathom, in their heart of hearts doctors usually know the real rationale for their actions. In the final analysis, each person must search his own conscience and decide whether or not to make financial arrangements that might compromise them. At issue is whether the public can trust us not only to be at their side, but on their side. Our collective actions will determine what our profession is to become, and I believe that most people are eager to attain the highest standards. Most people become physicians out of noble intentions. But as John Stuart Mill said, the capacity for noble feelings is a "very tender plant, easily killed, not by hostile influences, but by mere want of sustenance."[35] The profession is under siege by big business, and I do not perceive a vigorous effort to rescue it.

NOTES

Chapter 1

1. Vedantam, S. "Industry role in medical meeting decried. Symposium sponsored by pharmaceutical companies trouble some physicians." *Washington Post*, 2002 May 26; A10.
2. Reisman, R. E. Personal communication. 2001 Mar. 31.
3. Zaehringer, D. AllergyOne: Working Together as One for Optimal Allergy Treatment; 2004 Mar. 18.
4. Kesten, S. SPIRIVA HandiHaler Speaker Training, 2004 Apr. 1.
5. Kassirer, J. P., Harrington, J. T. "Diuretics and potassium metabolism. A reassessment of the need, effectiveness, and safety of potassium therapy." *Kidney International*, 1977; 11: 505–15.
6. Darves, B. "Too close for comfort? How some physicians are re-examining their dealings with drug detailers," *ACP Observer*, 2003 Jul./Aug.; 1, 13, 14.
7. Hensley, S. "AMA, Prescription-drug makers agree ethics policy needs better implementation," *Wall Street Journal*, 2002 Jan. 21; B4.
8. Holmer, A. F. "Industry strongly supports continuing medical education," *Journal of the American Medical Association*, 2001 Apr. 18; 285 (15): 2012–14.
9. *Recruitment News*, KL4-ARDS-04. Confidential Newsletter from Discovery Laboratories, Inc., 2002 Nov. 15.
10. "Gifts to physicians from industry." AMA, 2001. (Accessed Jan. 5, 2003, at www.ama-assn.org/ama/pub/article/4001-4236.html)
11. "PhRMA code on interactions with health-care professionals." In: *Pharmaceutical Research and Manufacturers of America*; 2002 Jul. 1; 1–9.
12. Grande, D., Volpp K. "Cost and quality of industry-sponsored meals for medical residents." *JAMA*, 2003; 290:1150–1.
13. Adams, C. "Doctors 'Dine 'n' Dash' in style, as drug firms pick up the tab," *Wall Street Journal*, 2001 May 14; 1.

14. Kassirer, J. P. "Financial indigestion." *JAMA*, 2000; 284 (17): 2156–57.
15. *U.S. v. TAP Pharmaceutical Products, Inc.*, No. 01-CR-10354-WGY (D. Mass. 2001).
16. Ibid.
17. Anonymous. Personal communication. 2002 Feb.
18. Stearns, N. S., Getchell, M. E., Gold, R. A. *Continuing medical education in community hospitals. A manual for program development.* Boston: Postgraduate Medical Institute, Massachusetts Medical Society; 1971.
19. Relman, A. S. "Defending professional independence: ACCME's proposed new guidelines for commercial support of CME." *JAMA*, 2003; 289 (18): 2418–20.
20. ACCME. List of ACCME-accredited providers. list; 2001 Sep. 5.
21. Letter to to [*sic*] the Accreditation Council for Graduate Medical Education regarding a Public Citizen study describing Medical Education Services Suppliers (HRG Publication # 1530). Public Citizen, 2001. (Accessed Dec. 13, 2001, at http://www.citizen.org/publications/release.cfm?ID=6731)
22. American Heart Association. Scientific sessions—satellite symposia; hard copies on file. *AHA*; Nov. 2002.
23. Campbell, E. G., Louis, K. S., Blumenthal, D. "Looking a gift horse in the mouth: corporate gifts supporting life sciences research." *JAMA*, 1998; 279 (13): 995–99.
24. Boyd, E. A., Bero, L. A. "Assessing faculty financial relationships with industry: a case study." *JAMA*, 2000; 284 (17): 2209–14.
25. Popeo, D. J., Samp, R. A. Comments of the Washington Legal Foundation to the Accreditation Council for Continuing Medical Education concerning request for comments on the 2003 Jan. 14 Draft "Standards to Ensure the Separation of Promotion From Education Within the CME Activities of ACCME Accredited Providers": Washington Legal Foundation; 2003 Jan. 29.
26. Society of American Gastrointestinal Endoscopic Surgeons. *SAGES 2003 Final Program.* Mar. 12–15; Los Angeles, CA.; 63–73.
27. Anonymous. Personal communication. 2001 Jan.
28. Angell, M., Kassirer, J. P. "Editorials and conflicts of interest." *New England Journal of Medicine*, 1996; 335 (14): 1055–56.
29. Knox, R. A. "At *NEJM*, clash over connections: New, old editors differ on conflict-of-interest regulations." *Boston Globe*, 2000 May 18; A1; Drazen, J. M., Curfman, G. D. "Financial associations of authors." *N Engl J Med*, 2002; 346 (24): 1901–02.
30. Keller, M. B., McCullough, J. P., Klein, D. N., et al. "A comparison of nefazodone, the cognitive behavioral-analysis system of psychotherapy, and their combination for the treatment of chronic depression." *N Engl J Med*, 2000; 342 (20): 1462–70.
31. Carpenter, C. C. J., Cooper, D. A., Fischl, M. A., et al. "Antiretroviral therapy in adults: updated recommendations of the International AIDS Society-USA Panel."

JAMA, 2000; 283 (3): 381–90; National Task Force on the Prevention & Treatment of Obesity. "Long-term pharmacotherapy in the management of obesity." *JAMA,* 1996; 276 (23): 1907–15.

32. "Emerging science of lipid management." *Lipid Letter,* 2002 Dec.: 2.
33. Cauchon, D. "FDA advisers tied to industry." *USA Today,* 2000 Sep. 25; 1A.
34. The Rezulin timeline. Saunders & Walker, Attorneys. (Accessed Oct. 22, 2003, at www.rezulin-updates.com/timeline.cfm)
35. Willman, D. "Stealth merger: Drug companies and government medical research." *Los Angeles Times,* 2003 Dec. 7.
36. Ibid.
37. Willman, D. "Probe sought into NIH officials' outside work. Three House Democrats ask the investigative arm of Congress to look into 'potential conflicts of interest' stemming from drug-firm payments." *Los Angeles Times,* 2004 Jan. 14.
38. Zirhouni, E. Letter to the Honorable W. J. "Billy" Tauzin, Chairman, Committee on Energy and Commerce, House of Representatives, Dec. 23, 2003.
39. Zirhouni, E. Memo to IC Directors, OD staff, NIH. Re: Awards, travel, and official duty and outside activity approvals - ACTION. Nov. 20, 2003.
40. Steinbrook, R. "Financial conflicts of interest and the NIH." *N Engl J Med,* 2004; 350: 327–30.
41. "The Integrity in Science Database: Scientists' & non-profits' ties to industry." The Center for Science in the Public Interest. (Accessed Jul. 31, 2003, at http://www.cspinet.org/integrity/database.html)

Chapter 2

1. Frizzell, L. "If you've got the money, honey, I've got the time": Columbia Records; 1950.
2. Armstrong, D., Zimmerman, R. "Pfizer settles Medicaid-fraud case for $430 million." *Wall Street Journal,* 2004 May 13.
3. Petersen, M. "Court papers suggest scale of drug's use: Lawsuit says doctors were paid endorsers." *New York Times,* 2003 May 30; C1.
4. McGough R., Callahan, P. "An illness that's not just for kids anymore." *Wall Street Journal,* 2003 Nov. 26; D1.
5. "Optimizing wakefulness in patients with fatigue and executive dysfunction." *The Primary Care Companion to the Journal of Clinical Psychiatry* 2003; 5 (Supplement 8).
6. Moore, T. J. "Cashing in on pain." *Washingtonian,* 2000 Jan. 31.
7. Wright, T. Flyer: "Achieving optimum outcomes: Customizing treatment for patients with HCV infection." In: *Education Initiative in Gastroenterology,* 2001.
8. Levin, J. Personal communication. 2001 Jan. 8.

9. Kramer, K. I. Letter to Boston academic physician, 2003 Mar. 12.

10. Faculty disclosure. *Managing HIT: Preventing life- and limb-threatening thrombosis.* Slide Kit. Presentation Manual: University of Pennsylvania School of Medicine; 2003 Apr. 26–27.

11. Anonymous. Personal communication. 2003 Mar. 23.

12. Ibid.

13. Agus, Z. S. Personal communication. 2003 Mar. 5, 11.

14. Petersen, M. "Madison Ave. has growing role in drug research." *New York Times,* 2002 Nov. 22; A1.

15. Giombetti, R. "Suicide science—Dr. David Dunner: Paxil's friendly ghostwriter?" 2002. (Accessed Aug. 22, 2002, at http://www.healthyskepticism.org)

16. "Prozac truth." (Accessed Aug. 22 , 2002, at http://www.prozactruth.com/fdalilly.htm); "Scandal of scientists who take money for papers ghostwritten by drug companies." *The Guardian,* 2002. (Accessed Jun. 24, 2002, at http://www.guardian.co.uk)

17. Kowalczyk, L. "Drug company push on doctors disclosed." *Boston Globe,* 2002 May 19; A1.

18. Brennan, T. A. "Buying editorials." *New England Journal of Medicine,* 1994; 331 (10): 673–5.

19. Petersen, M. "Madison Ave."

20. The AOA Mission. American Obesity Association, 2002. (Accessed Jul. 24, 2002, at www.obesity.org/subs/about.shtml)

21. Hurley, D. "Drugs may beat diets: Doctors; 2 medicines touted for obese." *Chicago Sun-Times,* 1994 Jun. 16; 12.

22. Johannes, L., Stecklow, S. "Dire warnings about obesity rely on slippery statistic." *Wall Street Journal,* 1998 Feb. 9; B1; The AOA Mission. American Obesity Association, 2002. (Accessed Jul. 24, 2002, at www.obesity.org/subs/about.shtml)

23. Advocacy update: Proposed approval of Xenical weight control drug. American Obesity Association, 1998. (Accessed Jul. 7, 2002, at www.obesity.org/subs/advocacy/FDA_Xenical.shtml)

24. "A taxpayer's guide on IRS policy to deduct weight control treatment." American Obesity Association, 2000. (Accessed Jul. 24, 2002, at www.online-xenical.com/irspolicy.html)

25. Johannes, L., Stecklow, S. "Dire warnings."

26. Atkinson, R. L. "Use of drugs in the treatment of obesity." *Annual Review of Nutrition,* 1997; 17: 383–403.

27. Kauffman, M., Julien, A. "Pushing a diet drug." *Hartford Courant,* 2000 Apr. 10.

28. Ibid.

29. The Integrity in Science Database. Scientists' & non-profits' ties to industry. The Center for Science in the Public Interest. (Accessed Jul. 31, 2003, at http://www.cspinet.org/integrity/database.html)

30. Johannes, L., Stecklow, S. "Dire warnings."

31. Abelson, R. "Drug sales bring huge profits, and scrutiny, to cancer doctors: Insurers and experts see high costs and conflicts." *New York Times*, 2003 Jan. 26; A1.; Alpert, B. "Hooked on drugs: Why do insurers pay such outrageous prices for pharmaceuticals?" *Barron's*, 1996 Jun. 10; 15.

32. Eisenberg, P. Personal communication. 2002 Oct. 20.

33. Greenwood, J. Joint hearing before the Subcommittee on Health and the Subcommittee on Oversight and Investigations. In: Committee on Energy and Commerce. 107th Congress, First Session ed. Washington DC: US Government Printing Office; 2001: 4.

34. Eisenberg, P.

35. Smith, T. J., Girtman, J., Riggins, J. "Why academic divisions of Hematology / Oncology are in trouble and some suggestions for resolution." *Journal of Clinical Oncology*, 2001; 19 (1): 260–64.

36. Harris, G. "Among cancer doctors, a Medicare revolt: New payment system spurs talk of return to hospital care and old drugs." *New York Times*, 2004 Mar. 11; C1.

37. Smith, T. J., Girtman, J., Riggins, J. "Why academic divisions."

38. Eisenberg, P.

39. Emanuel, E. J., Young-Xu, Y., Levinsky, N. G., Gazelle, G., Saynina, O., Ash, A. S. "Chemotherapy use among Medicare beneficiaries at the end of life." *Annals of Internal Medicine*, 2003; 138 (8): 639–43.

40. Harris, G. "Among cancer doctors."

41. Abelson, R. "Drug sales bring huge profits."

42. *U.S. v. TAP Pharmaceutical Products, Inc.*, No. 01-CR-10354-WGY (D. Mass. 2001).

43. Petersen, M. "2 drug makers to pay $875 million to settle fraud case." *New York Times,* 2001 Oct. 4.

44. *U.S. v. TAP Pharmaceutical Products, Inc.*

45. Ibid.

46. Ibid.

47. Petersen, M. "AstraZeneca pleads guilty in cancer medicine scheme: Taint of death doesn't slow marketing." *New York Times*, 2003 Jun. 22.

48. Fessenden, F., Drew, C. "Bottom line in mind, doctors sell Ephedra." *New York Times*, 2003 Mar. 31; A8.

49. Witlin, A. G., Mattar, F., Sabai, B. M. "Postpartum stroke: A twenty-year experience." *American Journal of Obstetrics and Gynecology*, 2000, 183: 83–8.

50. Witlin, A. Deposition, *Brasher v. Sandoz Pharmaceutical Corp.*; 1999 Jul. 28.

51. Sabai, B. M. Deposition, *Quinn v. Sandoz Pharmaceuticals Corp.*; 1999 Jul.11.

52. Witlin, A. Deposition.

53. Kristal, J. Letter to Frederick P. Zuspan, M.D. 1999 Aug. 6.

54. Ibid.
55. Brown v. American Home Products Corporation, 236 F. Supp. 2d 445 (E.D. Pa. 2002).
56. Ibid.
57. Ibid.
58. Willman, D. "The rise and fall of the killer drug Rezulin; people were dying as specialists waged war against their FDA superiors. Patient safety was at stake in the scramble to keep a 'fast-track' pill on the U.S. market, research reveals." *Los Angeles Times*, 2000 Jun. 4.
59. Willman, D. "Scientists who judged pill safety received fees; grants: Records show varied financial ties between researchers and maker of a diabetes drug linked to deaths." *Los Angeles Times*, 1999 Oct. 29.
60. Willman, D. "Drug maker hired NIH researcher; Rezulin: Doctor, superior deny any conflict of interest. Questions are raised about claims Warner-Lambert made in promoting the pill." Series: Second of two parts. *Los Angeles Times*, 1998 Dec. 7.
61. Willman, D. "National perspective; researcher's fees point to other potential conflicts at NIH; government's top expert on diabetes was paid by firm with stake in study he had role in. More 'questionable' payments surface." *Los Angeles Times*, 1999 Jan. 28.
62. Willman, D. "The rise and fall."
63. Ibid.
64. The Rezulin timeline. Saunders & Walker, Attorneys. (Accessed Oct. 22, 2003, at www.rezulin-updates.com/timeline.cfm)
65. Willman, D. "The rise and fall."
66. Pfizer Inc. 1st quarter report, form 10-Q: SEC; 2003 Mar. 30.
67. Willman, D. "The rise and fall."
68. Petersen, M. "Suit says company promoted drug in exam rooms." *New York Times*, 2002 May 15; C1.

Chapter 3

1. Thompson, D. F. "Understanding financial conflicts of interest." *New England Journal of Medicine* 1993, 329 (8): 573–76; Rodwin, M. A. *Medicine, money, & morals: Physicians' conflicts of interest.* New York: Oxford University Press, 1993; 8–9; Angell, M. "The doctor as double agent." *Kennedy Institute of Ethics Journal,* 1993; 3 (3): 279–86.
2. Malinowski, M. J. "Institutional conflicts and responsibilities in an age of academic-industry alliances." *Widener Law Symposium Journal,* 2001; 8 (1): 31–73.
3. McGinnis, J. M., Foege, W. H. "Actual causes of death in the United States." *Journal of the American Medical Association* 1993; 270: 2207–12.

4. Abenhaim, L., Moride Y., Brenot, F., et al. "Appetite-suppressant drugs and the risk of primary pulmonary hypertension." *N Engl J Med*,1996; 335 (9): 609–16.

5. Manson, J. E., Faich, G. A. "Pharmacotherapy for obesity—do the benefits outweigh the risks?" *N Engl J Med*, 1996; 335 (9): 659–60.

6. "Malpractice at medical journal?" *Boston Globe*, 1996 Sep. 1; D6.

7. Manson, J. E., Faich, G. A. "Pharmacotherapy for obesity."

8. Stark, A. *Conflict of interest in American public life*. Cambridge, MA: Harvard University Press, 2000; 241.

9. Ossorio, P. N. "Pills, bills and shills: Physician-researcher's conflicts of interest." *Widener Law Symposium Journal*, 2001; 8 (1): 75–103.

10. Davis, M. Introduction. In: Davis, M., Stark, A., eds. *Conflict of interest in the professions*. Oxford: Oxford University Press, 2001; 18.

11. Luban, D. "Law's blindfold." In: Davis, M., Stark, A., eds. *Conflict of interest in the professions*. Oxford: Oxford University Press, 2001; 23–48.

12. Grossman, W. Personal communication. 2003 Sep. 12.

13. Thompson, J., Baird, P., Downie, J. *The Olivieri Report*. Toronto: James Lorimer and Company, Ltd., 2001; 173.

14. Phillips, R. A., Hoey, J. "Constraints of interest: Lessons at the Hospital for Sick Children." *Canadian Medical Association Journal*, 1998; 159: 955–57.

15. Gibson, E., Baylis, F., Lewis, S. "Dances with the pharmaceutical industry." *CMAJ*, 2002; 166 (4): 448–50.

16. Ibid.

17. Smelser, N. Personal communication. 2002 May 2.

Chapter 4

1. Banks, J., Mainous, A. "Attitudes of medical school faculty toward gifts from the pharmaceutical industry." *Academic Medicine*, 1992; 69 (9): 610–12.

2. Waud, D. R. "Pharmaceutical promotions—a free lunch?" *New England Journal of Medicine*, 1992; 327 (5): 351–53.

3. Ende, M. "Pharmaceutical promotions." *N Engl J Med*, 1992; 327 (23): 1687.

4. Sobel, B. J. "Pharmaceutical promotions." *N Engl J Med*, 1992; 327 (23): 1686.

5. Anacker, A. "Pharmaceutical promotions." *N Engl J Med*, 1992; 327 (23): 1686.

6. Anonymous. Personal communication. 2002 Sep. 24.

7. Mattera, M. "Memo from the editor: Don't be the devil in the details." *Medical Economics*, 2002; 11: 4.

8. Noble, H. B. "Hailed as a Surgeon General, Koop criticized on web ethics." *New York Times*, 1999 Sep. 4.

9. Rizzoli, P. B. "View from the doctor's office." *Boston Globe*, 2002 Dec. 22; D10.

10. Murray, D. "Gifts: What's all the fuss about?" *Medical Economics*, 2002 Oct. 11: 119–20.

11. Barksdale, C. R. "Drug detailing." *ACP Observer,* 2003; 23 (9): 3.
12. Chren, M.-M., Landefeld, C. S. "Physicians' behavior and their interactions with drug companies: A controlled study of physicians who requested additions to a hospital drug formulary." *Journal of the American Medical Association,* 1994; 271 (9): 684–89.
13. Orlowski, J. P., Wateska, L. "The effects of pharmaceutical firm enticements on physician prescribing patterns: There's no such thing as a free lunch." *Chest,* 1992; 102 (1): 270–73.
14. Orlowski, J. P., Wateska, L. "The effects of pharmaceutical firm"; Wazana, A. "Physicians and the pharmaceutical industry: Is a gift ever just a gift?" *JAMA,* 2000; 283 (3): 373–80.
15. Cialdini, R. B. *Influence: Science and practice.* New York: Harper Collins College Publishers, 1993; 21.
16. Strohmetz, D. B., Rind, B., Fisher, R., Lynn, M. "Sweetening the till: The use of candy to increase restaurant tipping." *Journal of Applied Social Psychology,* 2002; 32: 300–09.
17. Goldfinger, S. "Sounding board: A matter of influence." *N Engl J Med,* 1987; 316 (22): 1408–09.
18. Katz, N. M. "How self-deception works." Unpublished manuscript 2003.
19. Steinman, M. A., Shlipak, M. G., McPhee, S. J. "Of principles and pens: Attitudes and practices of medicine housestaff toward pharmaceutical industry promotions." *American Journal of Medicine,* 2001; 110: 551–57.
20. Cappon, L. J., ed. *The Adams-Jefferson Letters: The Complete Correspondence Between Thomas Jefferson and Abigail and John Adams.* Chapel Hill: University of North Carolina, 1959.
21. Cialdini, R. B. *Influence: Science and practice.*
22. Smelser, N. Personal communication. 2002 May 2.
23. Anonymous. Personal communication. 2002 Nov. 7.
24. Anonymous nephrologist. Personal communication. 2003 May 5.
25. Gardner, H., Csikszentmihalyi, M., Damon, W. *Good work: When excellence and ethics meet.* New York: Basic Books, 2001.
26. Anonymous. Personal communication. 2002 Sep. 24.
27. Toffler, B. L., Reingold, J. *Final accounting: Ambition, greed, and the fall of Arthur Andersen.* New York: Broadway Books, 2003; 245.
28. Kerber, R. "Device makers target consumers with their ads." *Boston Globe,* 2004 Mar. 10; C1.
29. *Occupational Outlook Handbook: Physicians and surgeons.* Bureau of Labor Statistics, U.S. Department of Labor, 2003. (Accessed Sep. 27, 2003, at www.bls.gov/oco/ocos074.htm)

Chapter 5

1. Stelfox, H. T., Chua, G., O'Rourke, K., Detsky, A. S. "Conflict of interest in the debate over calcium-channel antagonists." *New England Journal of Medicine*, 1998; 338 (2): 101–06.
2. Smith, R. "Making progress with competing interests." *British Medical Journal*, 2002; 325: 1375–76.
3. Wennberg, J. E. "Dealing with medical practice variations: A proposal for action." *Health Affairs*, 2002 Mar. 6: 6–32.
4. Ibid.
5. Institute of Medicine. *Guidelines for clinical practice: From development to use.* Washington, DC: National Academy Press; 1992.
6. Shiffman, R. N., Shekelle, P., Overhage, J. M., Slutsky, J., Grimshaw, J., Deshpande, A. "Standardized reporting of clinical practice guidelines: A proposal from the conference on guideline standardization." *Annals of Internal Medicine*, 2003; 139 (6): 493–98.
7. Steinberg, E. P. "Improving the quality of care—can we practice what we preach?" *N Engl J Med*, 2003; 348 (26): 2681–83; Executive team. Resolution Health, Inc., 2003. (Accessed Jun. 30, 2003, at www.resolutionhealth.com)
8. Saag, M. "Is it time to proactively switch successful antiretroviral therapy? Carefully check your SWATCH." *Ann Intern Med*, 2003; 139 (2): 148–49.
9. Abraham, E., Reinhart, K., Opal, S., et al. "Efficacy and safety of tifacogin (recombinant tissue factor pathway inhibitor) in severe sepsis; a randomized controlled trial." *Journal of the American Medical Association*, 2003; 290 (2): 238–47.
10. Angus, D. C., Crowther, M. A. "Unraveling severe sepsis: Why did OPTIMIST fail and what's next?" *JAMA*, 2003; 290 (2): 256–58.
11. Warren, H. S., Suffredini, A. F., Eichacker, P. Q., Munford, R. S. "Risks and benefits of activated protein C treatment for severe sepsis." *N Engl J Med*, 2002; 347 (13): 1027–30.
12. Anonymous. Personal communication. 2003 Jul. 29.
13. Desnick, R. J., Brady, R., Barranger, J., et al. "Fabry Disease, an under-recognized multisystemic disorder: Expert recommendations for diagnosis, management, and enzyme replacement therapy." *Ann Intern Med*, 2003; 138 (4): 338–46.
14. Anonymous. Personal communication. 2003 Aug. 7.
15. Smith, R. "Medical journals and pharmaceutical companies: Uneasy bedfellows." *British Medical Journal*, 2003; 326: 1202–05.
16. Wilkes, M. S., Doblin, B. H., Shapiro, M. F. "Pharmaceutical advertisements in leading medical journals: Experts' assessments." *Ann Intern Med*, 1992; 116 (11): 912–19.

17. Landefeld, C. S., Chren, M.-M., Quinn, L. M., Siddique, R. M. "A 4-year study of the volume of drug advertisements in leading medical journals (abstract)." *Journal of General Internal Medicine*, 1995; 10 (Supplement):111.

18. Herman, J. G. Personal communication. 2003 Dec. 22.

19. Blackstone, T. S. Personal communication. 2004 Jan. 27.

20. Dyer, O. "Journal rejects article after objections from marketing department." *BMJ*, 2004; 328: 244.

21. Carver, D. Personal communication. 2004 Jan. 20.

22. Letter to to [*sic*] the Accreditation Council for Graduate Medical Education regarding a Public Citizen study describing Medical Education Services Suppliers (Publication # 1530). Public Citizen, 2001. (Accessed Dec. 13, 2001, at http://www.citizen.org/publications/release.cfm?ID=6731)

23. Relman, A. S. "Separating continuing medical education from pharmaceutical marketing." *JAMA*, 2001; 285 (15): 2009–12.

24. "Science for sale?" Transcript. *Now: With Bill Moyers*. Public Broadcasting Service. (Accessed Nov. 29, 2002, at www.pbs.org/now.printable/transcript_science forsale_print.html)

25. Relman, A. S. "Separating continuing medical education"; Holmer, A. F. "Industry strongly supports continuing medical education." *JAMA*, 2001; 285 (15): 2012–14.

26. Vergano, D. "Who's teaching the doctors? Drug firms sponsor required courses— and see their sales rise." *USA Today*, 2000 Mar. 9.

27. McDade, P. "Health care and pharmaceuticals." In: Hill & Knowlton Global. Worldwide Practices. Health Care and Pharmaceuticals 2001. (Accessed Nov. 26, 2001, at http://www.hillandknowlton.com/index.php?section1=practices& section2=health)

28. "Who we are." *Thomson Physicians World* (Accessed Jul. 31, 2003, at http:// www.physiciansworld.com/index2.asp?flash=no)

29. Relman, A. S. "Separating continuing medical education."

30. Vergano, D. "Who's teaching the doctors?"

31. Bowman, M. A. "The impact of drug company funding on the content of continuing medical education." *Mobius*, 1986; 6 (1): 66–69.

32. Bowman, M. A., Pearle, D. L. "Changes in drug prescribing patterns related to commercial company funding of continuing medical education." *Journal of Continuing Education in the Health Professions* 1988; 8: 13–20.

33. "About IFFGD." International Foundation for Functional Gastrointestinal Disorders, 2003. (Accessed Sep. 14, 2003, at www.iffgd.org/About/About.html)

34. Norton, N. Personal communication. 2003 Oct. 1.

35. "Rome I, Rome II, Rome III, and the Rome Committees: Terminology and bibliography." (Accessed Sep. 15, 2003, at www.romecriteria.org/rome12biolio.htm)

36. Drossman, D. A. Personal communication. 2003 Sep. 23.

37. "Disclosure of faculty relationships." In: 5th International Symposium on Functional Gastrointestinal Disorders; Apr. 4–7; 2003.

38. "Glaxo Wellcome decides to withdraw Lotronex from the market." U.S. Food and Drug Administration, 2000. (Accessed Oct. 27, 2003, at http://www.fda.gov/bbs/topics/ANSWERS/ANS01058.html)

39. Drossman, D. A. Editor's column: "Working in the FGID's, and the benefits and challenges of collaboration with industry." *Functional Brain-Gut Research Group Newsletter,* 2000 (24): 2.

40. "Disclosure of faculty relationships." In: 5th International Symposium on Functional Gastrointestinal Disorders; Apr. 4–7; 2003.

41. "Emerging Science of Lipid Management." *Lipid Letter,* 2002 Oct.

42. Ibid.

43. Editorial Board: Lipids Online. (Accessed Dec. 6, 2002, at http://www.lipids online.org/site/editorial.cfm)

44. Lipid Management: National Lipid Education Council; 2002/2003 Winter.

45. Libby P. Personal communication. 2003 Aug. 14.

46. "About NISE." National Initiative in Sepsis Education, 2002. (Accessed Dec. 5, 2002, at http://nise.cc/about.php3)

47. Moore, D. Personal communication. 2003 Sep. 4.

48. "Anemia: A hidden epidemic." National Anemia Action Council. Los Angeles: HealthVizion Communications Inc.; 2002.

49. AnemiaAlert: The E-newsletter of the National Anemia Action Council. Vol. 1, Number 5, October 2003; AnemiaAlert: The E-newsletter of the National Anemia Action Council. Vol.1, Number 6, December 2003.

50. Kleinschmidt, K., Miller, A., Pollack, C., Bosker, G. *Quick consult: Guide to clinical trials in thrombosis management.* 2d ed. Atlanta: American Health Consultants, 2002; 452.

51. Council for Leadership on Thrombosis. *Thrombosis crisis in hospital medicine and primary care.* April 26, 2003; Boston, MA: Thomson American Health Consultants; 2003.

52. Choudhry, N. K., Stelfox, H. T., Detsky, A. S. "Relationships between authors of clinical practice guidelines and the pharmaceutical industry." *JAMA,* 2002; 287 (5): 612–17.

Chapter 6

1. "Get complete access to the Endocrine Marketplace by partnering with the Endocrine Society." The Endocrine Society, 2002. (Accessed Sep. 16, 2002, at http://www.endo-society.org/industry/index.cfm)

2. Robertson, R. M. Personal communication. 2004 Apr. 15.

3. *Lifting the veil of secrecy: Corporate support for health and environmental professional associations, charities, and industry front groups.* Booklet. Washington, DC: Center for Science in the Public Interest; 2003 Jun.

4. "Corporate Advisory Council promotes education, research." *Academy News,* American Academy of Orthopaedic Surgeons, 2003. (Accessed Sep. 24, 2003, at www.aaos.org/wordhtml/2003news/a6-14.htm)

5. Antman, E. Personal communication. 2002 Jul. 28.

6. American Heart Association. "American Heart Association conflict of interest standards." In: *Policy and Procedure Manual.* AHA Scientific Publishing; 2003.

7. Antman, E.

8. "Guidelines 2000 for Cardiopulmonary Resuscitation and Emergency Cardiovascular Care." Supplement to *Circulation.* 2000; 102, Aug. 22.

9. Marler, J. for the National Institute of Neurological Disorders and Stroke rt-PA Stroke Study Group. "Tissue plasminogen activator for acute ischemic stroke." *New England Journal of Medicine,* 1995; 333: 1581–88.

10. Ibid.

11. Hoffman, J. R. "Should physicians give tPA to patients with acute ischemic stroke?" Against: "And just what is the emperor of stroke wearing?" *Western Journal of Medicine,* 2000; 173 (3): 149–50.

12. Bravata, D. M., Kim, N., Concato, J., Krumholz, H. M., Brass, L. M. Thrombolysis for acute stroke in routine clinical practice. *Archives of Internal Medicine,* 2002; 162: 1994–2001.

13. Lenzer, J. "Alteplase for stroke: Money and optimistic claims buttress the 'brain attack' campaign." *British Medical Journal,* 2002; 324: 723–29.

14. Ibid.

15. Faxon, D. "American Heart Association explains how guidelines were formulated." *British Medical Journal,* 2002; 324: 1581–82.

16. Mello, M. M., Studdert, D. M., Brennan, T. A. "The Leapfrog standards: Ready to jump from marketplace to courtroom?" *Health Affairs,* 2003; 22 (2): 45–59.

17. Peterson, E. Personal communication. 2002 Dec. 16.

18. CRUSADE Executive Committee. "A practical guide to understanding the 2002 ACC/AHA guidelines for the management of patients with non-ST-segment elevation acute coronary syndromes": Duke Clinical Research Institute; 2002 Jun.

19. "National Report from the Executive Committee of the CRUSADE National Quality Improvement Initiative." 2003. (Accessed Nov. 23, 2003, at www.crusadeqi.com/main/ecab/National_Report_Nov03.pdf)

20. "Drug that improves heart attack outcomes not used in 75 percent of patients." *Dukemed News,* 2003. (Accessed Oct. 15, 2003, at dukemednews.duke.edu); Linking quality of AMI care and outcomes. (Accessed Nov. 21, 2003, at http://www.hce.org/Medicare/Education/5_29_03Petersoncall.ppt)

21. CRUSADE Executive Committee. "A practical guide."

22. Peterson E. Personal communication. 2003 Jan. 20, 22, 24.

23. Freudenheim, M. "Panel says 3 allergy drugs should be sold over the counter." *New York Times*, 2001 May 12; B1; Lueck, S. "FDA considers unusual bid to end allergy drugs' prescription status." *Wall Street Journal*, 2001 May 11; B1.

24. Petersen, M. "Delays possible for over-the-counter allergy drugs." *New York Times*, 2001 May 16; C1–C7.

25. Harris, G. "Schering-Plough hurt by falling pill costs." *New York Times*, 2003 Jul. 8.

26. Petersen, M. "Delays possible for over-the-counter allergy drugs." *New York Times*, 2001 May 16; C1–C7; Petersen, M. "A push to sell top allergy drugs over the counter." *New York Times*, 2001 May 11; A1, C2.

27. Dr. Bob Lanier's Biography and current Curriculum Vitae. (Accessed Sep. 19, 2002, at askDrBob.com/bob.htm)

28. Kassirer, J. P., Reisman, R. E. "A prescription for industry control." *American Prospect*, 2001: 19.

29. Kassirer, J. P., Reisman, R. E. "A prescription for industry control"; Schatz, M. Letter from American Academy of Allergy, Asthma & Immunology to Fred Hassan, CEO of Schering-Plough Corporation. 2004 Apr. 14.

30. "Aventis Pharmaceuticals sales force voted #1 by Allergists." Flyer: *The Aventis Pharmaceuticals—AAAAI 2001 Partnership*, 2001, Aventis.

31. Kassirer, J. P., Reisman, R. E. "A prescription for industry control"; Speaker's bureau. American Academy of Allergy, Asthma and Immunology, 2002. (Accessed Sep. 19, 2002, at http://www.aaaai.org)

32. American Academy of Allergy Asthma and Immunology, 2002. 60th Anniversary Meeting—Sponsorship of meeting activities. (Accessed Sep. 19, 2002, at http://www.aaaai.org)

33. Petersen, M. "Pediatric book on breast-feeding stirs controversy with its cover." *New York Times*, 2002 Sep. 18; C1.

34. Ibid.

35. Ibid.

36. Gartner, L. M. Letter to Joe Sanders, Louis Cooper. 2002 Aug. 26.

37. Gartner, L. M. Personal communication. 2002 Sep. 22.

38. Sanders, J. M. Letter to Lawrence M. Gartner. 2002 Sep. 11.

39. American Thoracic Society. ATS 2002 Conference; Symposia excerpts. In: Ullman, K., ed., 2002; Atlanta, GA: Medical Association Communications, 2002.

40. Ibid.

41. Anonymous. Personal communication. 2002 Oct. 26.

42. Balk, R. A. Personal communication. 2002 Nov. 6.

43. American Thoracic Society. *ATS News*, 2002 Sep.

44. Winter, S. Personal communication. 2002 Oct. 2.

45. *Sponsorship opportunities.* 32nd Critical Care Congress, Society for Critical Care Medicine, San Antonio, Texas, Jan. 28–Feb. 2, 2003.

46. Ibid.

47. Harvey, M., Martin, D. J. Personal communication. 2002 Dec. 11.

48. "Corporate sponsorship opportunities." Digestive Disease Week, 2003. (Accessed Nov. 16, 2002, at www.ddw.org/exhibitors/sponsorshipopps.html)

49. *Nocturnal GERD.* CME booklet. Bethesda, MD: American Gastroenterological Association; 2002 Nov.

50. Stolar, M. Personal communication. 2002 Dec. 9, 13, 18.

51. *Nocturnal GERD.* CME booklet.

52. Groopman, J. "Hormones for men." *New Yorker,* 2002 Jul. 29.

53. Thorner, M., Buchner, D., Clemmons, D., et al. "Report of National Institute on Aging Advisory Panel on Testosterone Replacement in Men." *Journal of Clinical Endocrinology & Metabolism* 2001; 86 (10): 4611–14.

54. Groopman, J. "Hormones for men."

55. Bennett, W. Personal communication. 2003 Oct. 12.

56. Petersen, M. "Making drugs, shaping the rules." *New York Times,* 2004 Feb. 1.

57. Folstein, M. Personal communication. 2002 Aug. 8.

58. Nadelson, C. Personal communication. 2003 Sep. 4.

59. Cato, J. "Chester case may hinge on antidepressants. Report casts doubt on drug, suicide risk." *Rock Hill Herald,* 2004 Jan. 23; 1A.

60. Kendall, J. "Talking back to Prozac." *Boston Globe,* 2004 Feb. 1; H1; Harris, G. "Panel says Zoloft and cousins don't increase suicide risk." *New York Times,* 2004 Jan. 22; A12.

61. Cato, J. "Chester case may hinge on antidepressants. Report casts doubt on drug, suicide risk." *Rock Hill Herald,* 2004 Jan. 23; 1A.

62. Price, J. H. "Antidepressants, teen suicide link questioned." *Washington Times,* 2004 Feb. 8.

63. Romano, M. "Bittersweet. AMA reaps profits despite decreasing memberships." *Modern Healthcare,* 2003; 33 (22): 10.

64. Wolinsky, H., Brune, T. *The serpent on the staff: The unhealthy politics of the American Medical Association.* New York: G. P. Putnam's Sons, 1994; 15–43.

65. Kassirer, J. P., Angell, M. "The high price of product endorsement." *N Engl J Med,* 1997; 337 (10): 700.

66. Romano, M. "Prescription for conflict: AMA accepts funding from drug firms for campaign." *Modern Healthcare,* 2001 Jun. 18; Okie, S. "AMA blasted for letting drug firms pay for ethics campaign." *Washington Post,* 2001 Aug. 30; A3; Appleby, J. "Drugmakers bankroll ethics guidelines on 'freebies.'" *USA Today,* 2001 Apr. 27; 1B; Editorial. "An unhealthy influence on doctors." *New York Times,* 2001 Sep. 10; A28.

67. Krumholz, H. Personal communication. 2002 Dec. 16.

Chapter 7

1. Swartz, K., Brennan, T. A. "Integrated health care, capitated payment, and quality: The role of regulation." *Annals of Internal Medicine*, 1996; 124 (4): 442–48.
2. Managed care fact sheets: Managed care national statistics. Managed Care Online, 2003. (Accessed Nov. 15, 2003, at http://www.mcareol.com/factshts/factnati.htm)
3. Ritchie, J. Personal communication. 2003 Jun. 26.
4. Pollack, A. "California patients talk of needless heart surgery." *New York Times*, 2002 Nov. 4; C1; Wennberg, J. E., Fisher, E. S., Skinner, J. S. "Geography and the debate over Medicare reform." *Health Affairs*. Supp Web Exclusives:W96–114, 2002.
5. Maguire, P. "CT scans: New screening tool or risky fad?" *American College of Physicians Observer*, 2002 Feb.1.
6. Relman, A. S. "Dealing with conflicts of interest." *New England Journal of Medicine*, 1985; 313 (12): 749–51.
7. Ibid.
8. Morreim, E. H. "Unholy alliances: Physician investment for self-referral." *Radiology*, 1993; 186 (1): 67–72.
9. Hillman, B. J., Joseph, C. A., Mabry, M. R., Sunshine, J. H., Kennedy, S. D., Noether, M. "Frequency and costs of diagnostic imaging in office practice—a comparison of self-referring and radiologist-referring physicians." *N Engl J Med*, 1990; 323 (23): 1604–08.
10. Iglehart, J. K. "Efforts to address the problem of physician self-referral." *N Engl J Med*, 1991; 325: 1820–24.
11. Stark, F. Letter on the recent regulations on Stark II/ The Physician Self-referral Laws. 2000. (Accessed Nov. 15, 2003, at www.house.gov/stark/stark2/stark2.html)
12. Chase, L. "CMS calls the Stark II final rule a commonsense approach to preventing potentially abusive referrals while recognizing many legitimate financial arrangements." *Healthcare Financial Management*, Oct. 2001: 53–59; Chase, L. "The Stark II regulations: An analysis." *Western Journal of Medicine*, 2001; 175: 263–65; Melvin, D. H., Polacheck, J. F. "The final Stark II: Implications for hospital-physician arrangements." *Healthcare Financial Management*, Oct. 2001: 62–65.
13. Clancy, C. M., Brody, H. "Managed care: Jekyll or Hyde?" *Journal of the American Medical Association*, 1995; 273 (4): 338–39.
14. Kowalczyk, L. "Insurer tightening use of imaging tests." *Boston Globe*, 2004 Feb. 27; A1.
15. Armour, B. S., Pitts, M. M., Maclean, R., et al. "The effect of explicit financial incentives on physician behavior." *Archives of Internal Medicine*, 2001; 161: 1261–66.

16. Hillman, A. L., Pauly, M. V., Kerstein, J. J. "How do financial incentives affect physicians' clinical decisions and the financial performance of health maintenance organizations? [comment]. " *N Engl J Med*, 1989; 321 (2): 86–92.

17. Berwick, D. M. "Payment by capitation and the quality of care." *N Engl J Med*, 1996; 335 (16): 1227–31.

18. Wynia, M. K., VanGeest, J. B., Cummins, D. S., Wilson, I. B. "Do physicians not offer useful services because of coverage restrictions?" *Health Affairs*, 2003; 22 (4): 190–97.

19. Kerr, V. Personal communication. 2003 Jun. 27.

20. Feldman, D. S., Novack, D. H., Gracely, E. "Effects of managed care on physician-patient relationships, quality of care, and the ethical practice of medicine." *Arch Intern Med*, 1998; 158 (15): 1626–32.

21. Levinsky, N. G. "The doctor's master." *N Engl J Med*, 1984; 311: 1573–75; Angell, M. "The doctor as double agent." *Kennedy Institute of Ethics Journal*, 1993; 3 (3): 279–86; Kassirer, J. P. "Managed care and the morality of the marketplace." *N Engl J Med*, 1995; 331 (1): 50–52.

22. Woolhandler, S., Himmelstein, D. U. "Extreme risk—the new corporate proposition for physicians." *N Engl J Med*, 1995; 333: 1706–08.

23. Kassirer, J. P. "Managing care—should we adopt a new ethic?" *N Engl J Med*, 1998; 339 (6): 397–98.

24. Levinsky, N. G. "The doctor's master"; Angell, M. "The doctor as double agent." *Kennedy Institute of Ethics Journal*, 1993; 3 (3): 279–86; Kassirer, J. P. "Managing care—should we adopt a new ethic?" *N Engl J Med*, 1998; 339 (6): 397–98.

25. Levinson, W. "Paid not to refer?" *Journal of General Internal Medicine*, 2001; 16 (3): 209–10.

26. Mariner, W. K. "What recourse?—Liability for managed-care decisions and the Employee Retirement Income Security Act." *N Engl J Med*, 2000; 343 (8): 592–96.

27. Hammer, P. J. "Pegram v. Herdrich: On peritonitis, preemption, and the elusive goal of managed care accountability." *Journal of Health Politics, Policy & Law*, 2001; 26 (4): 767–87; *Pegram v. Herdrich*, 530 U.S. 211 (2000).

28. Mariner, W. K. "What recourse?"

29. *Pegram v. Herdrich*, 530 U.S. 211 (2000).

30. Hall, M. A. "Law, medicine, and trust." *Stanford Law Review*, 2002; 55: 463–527.

31. Gallagher, T. H., St. Peter, R., F., Chesney, M., Lo, B. "Patients' attitudes toward cost control bonuses for managed care physicians." *Health Affairs*, 2001; 20 (2): 186–92.

32. Garg, P. P., Frick, K. D., Diener-West, M., Powe, N. R. "Effect of the ownership of dialysis facilities on patients' survival and referral for transplantation." *N Engl J Med*, 1999; 341 (22): 1653–60.

33. Meyer, K. B., Kassirer, J. P. "Squeezing more cost and care out of dialysis: Our patients would pay the price." *American Journal of Medicine*, 2002; 112 (3): 232–34.

34. Ibid.

35. Garg, P. P., Frick, K. D., Diener-West, M., Powe, N. R. "Effect of the ownership"; Port, F. K., Wolfe, R. A., Held, P. J. "Ownership of dialysis facilities and patients' survival." *N Engl J Med*, 2000; 342 (14): 1053–56.

36. Klaidman, S. *Saving the heart: The battle to conquer coronary disease.* New York: Oxford University Press, 2000; 184–98.

37. Eichenwald, K., Kolata, G. "When physicians double as entrepreneurs." *New York Times*, 1999 Nov. 30; A1.

38. Herndon, J. Personal communication. 2003 Sep. 24.

39. Code of medical ethics and professionalism for orthopaedic surgeons. American Academy of Orthopaedic Surgeons, 2002. (Accessed Nov. 15, 2003, at www.aaos.org/wordhtml/papers/ethics/code.htm)

40. Miller, T. E., Sage, W. M. "Disclosing physician financial incentives." *JAMA*, 1999; 281 (15): 1424–30.

41. Hall, M. A., Kidd, K. E., Dugan, E. "Disclosure of physician incentives: Do practices satisfy purposes?" *Health Affairs*, 2000; 19 (4): 156–64; Miller, T. E., Horowitz, C. R. "Disclosing doctor's incentives: Will consumers understand and value the information?" *Health Affairs*, 2000; 19 (4): 149–55.

42. Hall, M. A. "Law, medicine, and trust." *Stanford Law Review*, 2002; 55: 463.

43. Miller, T. E., Horowitz, C. R. "Disclosing doctor's incentives: Will consumers understand and value the information?" *Health Affairs*, 2000; 19 (4): 149–55.

44. Epstein, A. M., Lee, T. H., Hamel, M. B. "Paying physicians for high-quality care." *N Engl J Med*, 2004; 350 (4): 406–10.

45. Kowalczyk, L. "For doctors, bonuses for quality care." *Boston Globe*, 2002 Nov. 7; A1

46. Epstein, A. M., Lee, T. H., Hamel, M. B. "Paying physicians for high-quality care." *N Engl J Med*, 2004; 350 (4): 406–10; Kowalczyk, L. "For doctors, bonuses for quality care." *Boston Globe*, 2002 Nov. 7; A1; Maguire, P. "California's new bonus programs: Good news for doctors?" *ACP Observer*, 2003 Mar.

47. Gold, M. R. "Financial incentives: Current realities and challenges for physicians." *J Gen Intern Med*, 1999; 14 (Supplement 1): s6–s12.

48. Hall, M. A., Berenson, R. A. "Ethical practice in managed care: A dose of realism." *Ann Intern Med*, 1998; 128 (5): 395–402.

Chapter 8

1. "National healthcare expenditures by type of service." Modern Healthcare, 2001. (Accessed Sep. 25, 2003, at http://nih.gov/about/);"FDA to speed up DTC regulatory actions: Investigators concerned that DTC ads drive medication use." *Formulary*, 2003; 38 (2): 115.

2. Bekelman, J. E., Li, Y., Gross, C. P. "Scope and impact of financial conflicts of interest in biomedical research: A systematic review." *Journal of the American Medical Association*, 2003; 289 (4): 454–65.

3. "Academia, industry, and the Bayh-Dole Act: An implied duty to commercialize." Unpublished manuscript. Center for Integration of Medicine and Innovative Technology (CIMIT), 2002. (Accessed Nov. 15, 2003, at www.cimit.org/coi_part3.pdf); Shaw, G. "Does the gene patenting stampede threaten science?" *Association of American Medical Colleges Reporter*, 2000; 9 (5). (Accessed Jul. 27, 2000, at www.aamc.org/newsroom/reporter/feb2000/gene.htm)

4. "Academia, industry, and the Bayh-Dole Act."

5. Relman, A. S. "The new medical-industrial complex." *New England Journal of Medicine*, 1980; 303 (17): 963–70.

6. "Academia, industry, and the Bayh-Dole Act"; Shaw, G. "Does the gene patenting stampede threaten science?" *Association of American Medical Colleges Reporter*, 2000; 9 (5). (Accessed Jul. 27, 2000, at www.aamc.org/newsroom/reporter/feb2000/gene.htm)

7. Kassirer, J. P. "More responsible medical leadership." *Boston Globe*, 2001 Feb. 17; A23.

8. Association of American Medical Colleges (AAMC), Task Force on Financial Conflicts of Interest in Clinical Research. *Protecting subjects, preserving trust, promoting progress I: Policy and guidelines for the oversight of individual financial interests in human subjects research.* 2001 Dec; Association of American Medical Colleges, Task Force on Financial Conflicts of Interest in Clinical Research. *Protecting subjects, preserving trust, promoting progress II: Principles and recommendations for oversight of an institution's financial interests in human subjects research.* 2002 Oct.; Fleetwood, J. "Conflicts of interest in clinical research: Advocating for patient-subjects." *Widener Law Symposium Journal*, 2001; 8 (1): 105–14; Moses, H., Braunwald, E., Martin, J. B., Thier, S. O. "Collaborating with industry—choices for the academic medical center." *N Engl J Med*, 2002; 347 (17): 1371–75.

9. Washburn, J. "Informed consent: Alan Milstein says he wants to rescue us from unscrupulous doctors, undisclosed risks and greedy institutions. But is he a shining knight, or an enemy of medical progress?" *Washington Post*, 2001 Dec. 30; W16.

10. Ibid.

11. Ibid.

12. Ibid.

13. Ibid.

14. Ibid.

15. Nelson, D., Weiss, R. "Hasty Decisions in race to a cure?" *Washington Post*, 1999 Nov. 21; A1.

16. Dembner, A. "Wrongful-death suit asserts gene therapy facts withheld." *Boston Globe*, 2002 May 18; B1; Dembner, A., Kowalczyk, L. "Doctor stirs questions on genetics' frontier." *Boston Globe*, 2000 May 21; A1.

17. Ibid.

18. Ibid.

19. Eichenwald, K., Kolata, G. "When physicians double as entrepreneurs." *New York Times*, 1999 Nov. 30; A1.

20. Nelson, D., Weiss, R. "FDA stops researcher's human gene therapy experiments." *Washington Post*, 2000 Mar. 2; A8.

21. Wilson, D., Heath, D. "Uninformed consent. A five-part *Seattle Times* investigative series." *Seattle Times*, 2001 Mar. 11–15; 1–15.

22. Ibid.

23. Heath, D., Timmerman, L. "Jury finds Hutch not negligent in 4 deaths." *Seattle Times*, 2004 Apr. 9.

24. Fred Hutchinson Cancer Research Center Board of Trustees. Patient Protection Oversight Committee Progress Report; 2002 Apr. 25.

25. Cho, M. K., Shohara, R., Schissel, A., Rennie, D. "Policies on faculty conflicts of interest at US universities." *JAMA*, 2000; 284 (17): 2203–08.

26. Korn, D. "Conflicts of interest in biomedical research." *JAMA*, 2000; 284 (17): 2234–37.

27. Eichenwald, K., Kolata, G. "Research for hire: Drug trials hide conflicts for doctors." *New York Times*, 1999 May 16; 1.

28. Bodenheimer. T. "Uneasy alliance: Clinical investigators and the pharmaceutical industry." *N Engl J Med*, 2000; 342 (20): 1539–44.

29. Eichenwald, K., Kolata, G. "Research for hire."

30. Ibid.

31. Ibid.

32. Ibid.

33. Bodenheimer. T. "Uneasy alliance."

34. Charatan, F. "US drug trials expand outside academic centres." *British Medical Journal*, 1999; 318: 1442.

35. Snyderman, R., Holmes, E. W. "Oversight mechanisms for clinical research." *Science*, 2000; 287: 595–97; Steinbrook, R. "Improving protection for research subjects." *N Engl J Med*, 2002; 346: 1425–30.

36. Office for Human Research Protections. *Draft interim guidance. Financial relationships in clinical research: Issues for institutions, clinical investigators, and IRBs to consider when dealing with issues of financial interest and human subject protection*, 2001 Jan. 10.

37. Malinowski, M. J. "Institutional conflicts and responsibilities in an age of academic-industry alliances." *Widener Law Symposium Journal*, 2001; 8 (1): 31–73.

38. McCrary, S. V., Anderson, C. B., Jakovljevic, J., et al. "A national survey of policies on disclosure of conflicts of interest in biomedical research." *N Engl J Med*, 2000; 343 (22): 1621–26.

39. Lo, B., Wolf, L. E., Berkeley, A. "Conflict-of-interest policies for investigators in clinical trials." *N Engl J Med*, 2000; 343 (22): 1616–20.

40. Ossorio, P. N. "Pills, bills and shills: Physician-researcher's conflicts of interest." *Widener Law Symposium Journal*, 2001; 8 (1): 75–103.

41. AAMC. *promoting progress* I, *promoting progress* II.

42. Moses, H., Braunwald, E., Martin, J. B., Thier, S. O. "Collaborating with industry—choices for the academic medical center." *N Engl J Med*, 2002; 347 (17): 1371–75.

43. Dale, M. L. Personal communication. 2004 Jun. 9.

44. Ibid.

45. Relman, A. S., Angell, M. "America's other drug problem." *New Republic*, 2002 Dec. 16.

46. Nathan, D. G., Weatherall, D. J. "Academic freedom in clinical research." *N Engl J Med*, 2002; 347 (17): 1368–70.

47. Bodenheimer, T. "Uneasy alliance."

48. Bekelman, J. E., Li, Y., Gross, C. P. "Scope and impact of financial conflicts."

49. Bodenheimer, T. "Uneasy alliance."

50. Davidoff, F., DeAngelis, C. D., Drazen, J. M., et al. "Sponsorship, authorship, and accountability." *N Engl J Med*, 2001; 345 (11): 825–26.

51. Anonymous. "Publication ethics from the Uniform Requirements for Manuscripts Submitted to Biomedical Journals." *N Engl J Med*, 2001; 345: 826–27.

52. Bodenheimer, T. "Uneasy alliance."

53. Blumenthal, D., Campbell, E. G., Anderson, M. S., Causino, N., Louis, K. S. "Withholding research results in academic life science: Evidence from a national survey of faculty." *JAMA*, 1997; 277 (15): 1224–28.

54. Blumenthal, D., Causino, N., Campbell, E. G., Louis, K. S. "Relationships between academic institutions and industry in the life sciences—an industry survey." *N Engl J Med*, 1996; 334 (6): 368–73.

55. Davidson, R. A. "Source of funding and outcome of clinical trials." *J Gen Intern Med*, 1986; 1: 155–56; Friedberg, M. "Evaluation of conflict of interest in economic analyses of new drugs used in oncology." *JAMA*, 1999; 282: 1453–55; Smith, R. "Making progress with competing interests." *British Medical Journal*, 2002; 325: 1375–76.

56. Krimsky, S. *Science in the private interest: Has the lure of profits corrupted biomedical research?* Lanham, Maryland: Rowman and Littlefield, 2003.

Chapter 9

1. "The Doctor," 1891, by Sir Luke Fildes (1844–1927), Oil on canvas, 166.4 x 241.9 cm. Tate Gallery, London.

2. Anonymous. "Profits of medical practice." *Boston Medical and Surgical Journal*, 1847: 203.

3. O'Neill, E. *Long day's journey into night*. 2d ed. New Haven: Yale University Press, 2002; 27.

4. Ibid., 148–49.

5. Maurer, H. "The MD's are off their pedestal." *Fortune*, 1954 Feb.; 138.

6. Rothman, D. J. "Medical professionalism—focusing on the real issues." *New England Journal of Medicine*, 2000; 342 (17): 1284–86.

7. Kassirer, J. P. "Doctor discontent." *N Engl J Med*, 1998; 339 (21): 1543–45.

8. Behind the times: Physician income, 1995–1999. Mar. 2003. (Accessed Sep. 1, 2003, at http://www.hschange.com/CONTENT/544/)

9. Ludmerer, K. M. Personal communication. 2003 Nov. 20.

10. Stanford University Corporate Guide. Top 10 Stanford Inventions. Recombinant DNA Cloning Technology. 2003. (Accessed Sep. 1, 2002, at http://corporate.stanford.edu/innovations/invent.html)

11. Thursby, J. G., Thursby, M. C. "University licensing and the Bayh-Dole Act." *Science*, 2003; 301: 1052.

12. Thursby, J. G., Thursby, M. C. "University licensing and the Bayh-Dole Act"; Washburn, J., Press, E. "The Kept University." *Atlantic Monthly*, 2000 Mar.

13. Relman, A. S. "The new medical-industrial complex." *N Engl J Med*, 1980; 303 (17): 963–70.

14. Malinowski, M. J. "Institutional conflicts and responsibilities in an age of academic-industry alliances." *Widener Law Symposium Journal*, 2001; 8 (1): 31–73.

15. Kassirer, J. P. "Tribulations and rewards of academic medicine: Where does teaching fit?" *N Engl J Med*, 1996; 334: 184–85.

16. Ludmerer, K. M. "Internal malaise." In: *Time to heal: American medical education from the turn of the century to the era of managed care*. Oxford: Oxford University Press, 1999; 348.

17. Kassirer, J. P. "Medicine at center stage." *N Engl J Med*, 1993; 328: 1268–69.

18. Breen, S. "Things you can buy with your tax rebate check." *USA Today*, 2001 Jul. 24; 11A.

19. Barringer, F. "Ex-publisher assails paper in Los Angeles." *New York Times*, 1999 Nov. 4.

20. Jurkowitz, M. "*LA Times* details its Staples faults." *Boston Globe*, 1999 Dec. 21; D1.

21. Petersen, M. "CNN to reveal when guests promote drugs for companies." *New York Times*, 2002 Aug. 23; C1.

22. Kuczynski, A. "Treating disease with a famous face." *New York Times*, 2002 Dec. 15.
23. Morgenstern, G. "Buy, they say; but what do they do?" *New York Times*, 2001 May 27.
24. Johannes, L., Hechsinger, J. "Why a brokerage giant pushes some mediocre mutual funds." *Wall Street Journal*, 2004 Jan. 9; A1.
25. Pianin, E. "Toxic chemical review process faulted; scientists on EPA Advisory Panels often have conflicts of interest, GAO says." *Washington Post*, 2001 Jul. 16; A2.
26. Mikva, A. "The wooing of our judges." *New York Times*, 2000 Aug. 28.
27. Holland, G. "Chief justice orders examination of judicial ethics after Scalia issue." *Boston Globe*, 2004 May 26; A2.
28. Editorial. "Strengthening the rules for America's judges." *International Herald Tribune*, 2004 May 28; 8.
29. "Supreme Court Justice few folks can afford." Texans for Public Justice. (Accessed Jan. 6, 2002, at http://www.tpj.org/opeds/payola_oped.htm)
30. Greising, D. "'Chinese walls' are no match for temptation." *Chicago Tribune*, 2001 Nov. 4.
31. "Six crucial lessons of the Enron saga." *Wall Street Journal*, 2002. (Accessed Jun. 20, 2002, at http://www.msnbc.com/)
32. Eichenwald, K. "Audacious climb to success ended in a dizzying plunge." *New York Times*, 2002 Jan.13; 1.
33. Ridgeway, J. "Phil Gramm's Enron favor." *Village Voice*, 2002. (Accessed Jan. 16, 2002, at www.villagevoice.com/issues/0203/ridgeway.php)
34. Ridgeway, J. "Phil Gramm's Enron favor"; Gerth, J., Oppel, R. A. "Senate Bill showed complexities of power couple's ties to Enron." *New York Times*, 2002 Jan.18; C1.
35. Francis, D. R. "Executive-pay hikes raise ire of unions and others." *Christian Science Monitor*, 2003 Apr. 28; 17.
36. Lee, F. R. "In today's business world, can doing good also mean doing well?" *New York Times*, 2002 Oct. 19; A21.
37. Handy, C. "What's a business for?" *Harvard Business Review*, 2002 Dec.; 49–55.
38. Kassirer, J. P. "Medicine at the turn of the century." *Annals of Thoracic Surgery*, 2000; 70: 351–53.
39. Martin, D. "Salvator Altchek, 'the $5 Doctor,' of Brooklyn, dies at 92." *New York Times*, 2002 Sep. 15.

Chapter 10

1. *Sicily*. Melbourne: Lonely Planet Publishers; 2002.
2. Gaiter, D. J., Brecher, J. "Seizing Nouveau's moment." *Wall Street Journal*, 2003 Nov. 28; W7.

3. Thompson, D. F. "Understanding financial conflicts of interest." *New England Journal of Medicine*, 1993; 329 (8): 573–76; Rodwin, M. A. *Medicine, money, & morals: Physicians' conflicts of interest*. New York: Oxford University Press, 1993; 213–19.

4. Malinowski, M. J. "Institutional conflicts and responsibilities in an age of academic-industry alliances." *Widener Law Symposium Journal*, 2001; 8 (1): 31–73.

5. Thompson, D. F. "Understanding financial conflicts of interest"; Rodwin, M. A. "Physicians' conflicts of interest: The limitations of disclosure." *N Engl J Med*, 1989; 321 (20): 1405–08; Stark, A. *Conflict of interest in American public life*. Cambridge, MA: Harvard University Press, 2000; 241.

6. American Society of Hematology. "Disclosure index." In: *American Society of Hematology, Annual Meeting 2000*; 848a.

7. Surowiecki, J. "The talking cure." *New Yorker*, 2002 Dec. 9; 54.

8. Ibid.

9. Brennan, T. A. "Buying editorials." *N Engl J Med*, 1994; 331 (10): 673–75; Kassirer, J. P. "Financial conflict of interest: An unresolved ethical frontier." *American Journal of Law & Medicine*, 2001; 27 (2–3): 149–62.

10. AMA Council on Ethical and Judicial Affairs. "Guidelines on Gifts to Physicians From Industry: An Update." *Food and Drug Law Journal*, 2001; 56 (1): 27–40.

11. American College of Physicians. *Ethics Manual*. Fourth Edition. 1997–1998. (Accessed Sep. 2, 2003, at www.acponline.org/ethics/ethicman.htm#conflict.)

12. Sox, H. C. "Medical professionalism in the new millennium: A physician charter." *Annals of Internal Medicine*, 2002; 136 (3): 243–46.

13. American Bar Association. *Model Code of Judicial Conduct*, 2000; Canon 3E. (Accessed May 31, 2004, at http://www.abanet.org/cpr/mcjc/canon_3.html)

14. Clark, K. "Regulating the conflict of interest of government officials." In: Davis M., Stark, A., eds., *Conflict of interest in the professions*. Oxford: Oxford University Press, 2001; 49–70.

15. Rodwin, M. A. *Medicine, money, & morals*.

16. Clark, K. "Regulating the conflict of interest." Rodwin, M. A. *Medicine, money, & morals*.

17. Borden, S., Pritchard, M. "Conflict of interest in journalism." In: Davis, M., Stark, A., eds., *Conflict of interest in the professions*. Oxford: Oxford University Press, 2001; 73–91.

18. *Ethical journalism: Code of Conduct for the News and Editorial Departments*. New York: *New York Times*; 2003 Jan.

19. Petersen, M. "Vermont to require drug makers to disclose payments to doctors." *New York Times*, 2002 Jun. 13; C1.

20. Johannes, L. "Vermont to require drug companies to disclose gifts." *Wall Street Journal*, 2002 Jun. 14.

21. Kaufman, M. "Vt. requires firms to report gifts to doctors; law prompted by concern about abuses, cost of drug companies' marketing." *Washington Post*, 2002 Jun. 14; A2.

22. Maves, M. D. Letter to Janet Rehnquist, J.D., Inspector General. Department of Health and Human Services. In: Chicago; 2002 May 26.

23. Chimonas, S., Rothman, D. J. *Draft vs. Final OIG Compliance Program Guidance: Influence of the medical profession and the pharmaceutical industry.* Unpublished manuscript; 2003, 1–40.

24. Foubister, V. "Gene therapy group adopts stringent rules on financial ties." *American Medical News*, 2000; 10–11.

25. Association of American Medical Colleges (AAMC), Task Force on Financial Conflicts of Interest in Clinical Research. *Protecting subjects, preserving trust, promoting progress I: Policy and guidelines for the oversight of individual financial interests in human subjects research.* 2001 Dec.; Association of American Medical Colleges, Task Force on Financial Conflicts of Interest in Clinical Research. *Protecting subjects, preserving trust, promoting progress II: Principles and recommendations for oversight of an institution's financial interests in human subjects research.* 2002 Oct.

26. In May, 2004, the Department of Health and Human Services issued final guidance for researchers regarding human subject protection in institutional situations complicated by financial conflict of interest. Among the actions it recommended "considering," for federally funded research, was using individuals from outside the institution in the review and oversight of financial conflicts of interest. See: Department of Health and Human Services. Financial relationships and interests in research involving human subjects: guidance for human subject protection. Federal Register / Vol. 69, No. 92 / Wednesday, May 12, 2004 / Notices.

27. Department of Health and Human Services. Financial relationships and interests in research involving human subjects: guidance for human subject protection. Federal Register / Vol. 69, No. 92 / Wednesday, May 12, 2004 / Notices.

28. Kuhlik, B. Personal communication. 2004 Mar. 12.

29. Krugman, P. "Delusions of power." *New York Times*, 2003 Mar. 28; A19.

30. Borowitz, A. "George W. Bush, news junkie." *New Yorker*, 2003 Oct. 13; 46.

31. Waud, D. R. "Pharmaceutical promotions—a free lunch?" *N Engl J Med*, 1992; 327 (5): 351–53; Kassirer, J. P. "Financial conflict of interest: An unresolved ethical frontier." *American Journal of Law & Medicine*, 2001; 27 (2–3): 149–62; Relman, A. S. "Dealing with conflicts of interest." *N Engl J Med*, 1985; 313 (12): 749–51; Angell, M. "Is academic medicine for sale?" *N Engl J Med*, 2000; 342 (20): 1516–18; Rothman, D. J. "Medical professionalism—focusing on the real issues." *N Engl J Med*, 2000; 342 (17): 1284–86; Dana, J., Loewenstein, G. "A

social science perspective on gifts to physicians from industry." *JAMA*, 2003; 290 (2): 252–55.

32. AAMC. *promoting progress* I, *promoting progress* II; American Board of Internal Medicine. *ABIM conflict of interest and confidentiality policies.* 1997; Moses, H., Martin, J. B. "Academic relationships with industry: A new model for biomedical research." *JAMA*, 2001; 285 (7): 933–35; Moses, H., Braunwald, E., Martin, J. B., Thier, S. O. "Collaborating with industry—choices for the academic medical center." *N Engl J Med*, 2002; 347 (17): 1371–75.

33. Verma, S. "A Matter of Influence: Graduate Medical Education and Commercial Sponsorship." *N Engl J Med*, 1988; 318 (1): 52–53.

34. AMSA policy on pharmaceutical promotions. 2002. (Accessed Sep. 11, 2003, at http://www.amsa.org/prof/policy.cfm)

35. Mill, J. S. *Utilitarianism.* In: Adler, M. J., Fadiman, C., and Goetz, P., eds. *Great Books of the Western World.* 2nd ed. Chicago: Encyclopaedia Britannica,1990; 40: 449d.

INDEX